Becoming a Health Care Professional

Student Activity Guide

Sherry Makely, PhD, R.T.(R)
Shirley A. Badasch, M.Ed, RN
Doreen S. Chesebro, B.Ed, LVN

PEARSON

Boston   Columbus   Indianapolis   New York   San Francisco   Upper Saddle River
Amsterdam   Cape Town   Dubai   London   Madrid   Milan   Munich   Paris   Montreal   Toronto
Delhi   Mexico City   São Paulo   Sydney   Hong Kong   Seoul   Singapore   Taipei   Tokyo

10 9 8 7 6 5 4 3 2 1

PEARSON

ISBN 10:   0-13-284338-2
ISBN 13: 978-0-13-284338-6

Contents

Introduction to the Student Activity Guide

The *Student Activity Guide* is a supplement to the textbook *Becoming a Health Care Professional, First Edition.* Aligned with each section in the textbook, the *Student Activity Guide* presents more than one hundred different learning activities. These learning activities are designed to help you strengthen your critical-thinking skills and review and apply what you are learning through your textbook reading assignments.

To use the *Student Activity Guide* most effectively:

- Review the section objectives. Each objective tells you what you are expected to learn and to know by the end of the section.

- Follow the directions. Complete each worksheet as instructed and assigned by your teacher. Use extra sheets of paper when needed to record your answers.

- Use extra sheets of paper or the Notes pages at the back of your book when needed to record your answers.

- Use your textbook to help you complete the worksheets. Some of the worksheets will help you review information in the textbook while others will help you continue your learning.

- Think about how to apply what you're learning. As an alternative to memorization and recall, worksheets are designed to stimulate and develop your critical-thinking skills.

- Complete the worksheets in the order in which they are presented. Each worksheet builds on another, so do not move on until you are certain that you have completed all worksheets to the best of your ability.

- Work as an individual or as part of a team. Some worksheets are designed for you to complete on your own. Other worksheets call for a team effort with your classmates and teacher.

- Expect to spend some time completing the assignments. Some of the worksheets can be completed relatively quickly while others will require significantly more time.

- Develop your research skills. Several worksheets require some research on your part. Learning how to access and use references such as Internet websites and library resources to find the information you need is an essential part of your education.

- Undergo an evaluation. When you have completed each worksheet and are confident that you can meet the objectives listed, ask your teacher for the section evaluation. The section evaluation is one method to measure your mastery of the material presented.

Once you have completed your textbook reading assignments and the worksheets in this *Student Activity Guide* you will be well on your way to becoming a health care professional.

Enjoy the journey!

Chapter 1 • Introduction to Health Careers
Section 1.1 Professionalism in Health Care

■ Objectives

After completing this section, you will be able to:

1. Define the key terms.
2. Explain why professionalism is important in health care.
3. List the characteristics that define a *health care professional*.
4. Describe how to identify a health care professional when you see one.
5. Explain the statement, "It's not the job you do that makes you a professional, it's how you do your job that counts."
6. Discuss the impact that a successful health career can have on your self-esteem and self-worth.
7. Explain why health care workers need an attitude that supports service to others.
8. List five steps you can take now to begin developing your professional reputation.

■ Directions

1. Read Section 1.1 in your textbook.
2. Complete Worksheet 1.
3. Complete Worksheet 2.
4. Complete Worksheet 3.
5. Complete Worksheet 4.

■ Evaluation Method

- Worksheets
- Class participation
- Section test

Professionalism in Health Care

1. List three types of health care workers whose jobs require professionalism. Give one reason why professionalism is important in each job.

Job	Why professionalism is important
Example:	
Doctor	The wrong diagnosis could harm the patient
1. _____	_____
2. _____	_____
3. _____	_____

2. Which of the following health care workers have the opportunity to be recognized by other people as a health care professional? Circle each correct answer.

   A. housekeepers

   B. pharmacy technicians

   C. purchasing agents

   D. radiographers

   E. nurses

   F. medical secretaries

   G. medical assistants

   H. laundry workers

   I. surgical technologists

   Write a brief paragraph to explain your answer:

3. List three characteristics that define a *health care professional*:

   1. _____

   2. _____

   3. _____

■ Worksheet 2

Recognition as a Health Care Professional

Make two lists. In list #1, identify five things that a health care worker *should do* to be seen by others as a professional. In list #2, identify five things that a health care worker *should not do* to avoid being seen as unprofessional.

List #1 "Should Do"

1. _____
2. _____
3. _____
4. _____
5. _____

List #2 "Should Not Do"

1. _____
2. _____
3. _____
4. _____
5. _____

■ **Worksheet 3**

My Professional Reputation Plan

Create a written plan to begin developing your professional reputation now. In the space below, state three goals that you need to achieve. Goal #1 should be the most important, followed by Goal #2, etc.

Goal #1 _____

Goal #2 _____

Goal #3 _____

Starting with Goal #1, list the steps you will take to achieve your goal. Identify the resources you will need and describe how you will obtain them. List any barriers that you might encounter and your plans to overcome them.

Goal #1

    Steps I will take:

    Resources I will need:

    Barriers and plans to overcome them:

Goal #2

    Steps I will take:

    Resources I will need:

    Barriers and plans to overcome them:

Goal #3

    Steps I will take:

    Resources I will need:

    Barriers and plans to overcome them:

■ Worksheet 4

Matching Key Terms with Definitions

Key Terms #1: Match each term with its correct definition:

_____ 1. accreditation

_____ 2. attitude

_____ 3. caregivers

_____ 4. certifications

_____ 5. competence

_____ 6. credentials

_____ 7. cultures

_____ 8. diagnostic

_____ 9. dignity

_____ 10. ethics

a. letters or certificates given to a person to show that he or she has the right to exercise a certain authority

b. a manner of acting, feeling, or thinking that shows one's disposition or opinion

c. health care workers who provide direct, hands-on patient care

d. possessing necessary knowledge and skills

e. certified as having met set standards

f. credentials from a state agency or a professional association awarding permission to use a special professional title; must meet pre-established competency standards

g. the degree of worth, merit, honor

h. having precedence in time, order, and importance

i. groups of people who share the same values, norms, and behaviors

j. deciding the nature of a disease or condition

k. standards of conduct and moral judgment

Key Terms #2: Match each term with its correct definition:

_____ 1. GED

_____ 2. goals

_____ 3. hierarchy

_____ 4. internship

_____ 5. licenses

_____ 6. payers

_____ 7. postsecondary

_____ 8. priorities

_____ 9. professional associations

_____ 10. professionals

_____ 11. credible

a. a real-life learning experience obtained through working on-site in a health care facility while enrolled as a student

b. a group of people or units arranged by rank

c. a high school equivalency credential

d. credentials from a state agency awarding legal permission to practice; must meet pre-established qualifications

e. someone that covers the expense for goods received or services rendered

f. after high school

g. aim, objects, or ends that one strives to attain

h. having precedence in time, order, and importance

i. people with experience and skills who are engaged in a specific occupation for pay or as a means of livelihood

j. worthy of being trusted and believed

k. organizations composed of people from the same occupation

l. standards of conduct and moral judgment

Key Terms #3: Match each term with its correct definition:

_____ 1. providers

_____ 2. reputation

_____ 3. respect

_____ 4. scope of practice

_____ 5. self-esteem

_____ 6. self-worth

_____ 7. socioeconomic status

_____ 8. therapeutic

_____ 9. trust

_____ 10. vendors

_____ 11. traits

a. belief in oneself, self-respect

b. importance and value in oneself

c. social rank in a community based on income, education, occupation, and so forth

d. treating or curing a disease or condition

e. to place confidence in the honesty, integrity, and reliability of another person

f. people who work for companies with which your company does business

g. boundaries that determine what a worker may and may not do as part of his or her job

h. feeling or showing honor or esteem

i. personality characteristics

j. a person's character, values, and behavior as viewed by others

k. doctors, health care workers, and health care organizations that offer health care services

l. aim, objects, or ends that one strives to attain

Section 1.2 Overview of Health Careers

■ Objectives

After completing this section, you will be able to:

1. Define the key terms.
2. Describe the purpose of the National Career Clusters™ Framework.
3. List three of the sixteen Career Clusters in addition to Health Science.
4. List the five Health Science pathways.
5. Describe the purpose of the National Consortium for Health Science Education.
6. Name three of the eleven foundation standards topics covered by the National Healthcare Skills Standards.
7. Describe the role that each of the following plays in health care: Therapeutic Services, Diagnostic Services, Health Informatics Services, Support Services, and Biotechnology Research and Development Services.
8. Name one health occupation for each of the five Health Science service areas.
9. Name two health occupations aligned with systems of the human body.
10. Name two careers in alternative health services.
11. Name two careers in medicine.

■ Directions

1. Read Section 1.2 in your textbook.
2. Complete Worksheets 1 and 2.
3. With your teacher's help, complete Worksheet 3.
4. Complete Worksheet 4.

■ Evaluation Method

- Worksheets
- Class participation
- Section test

■ Worksheet 1

Health Service Areas

Compare the services performed by the diagnostic, therapeutic, informatics, support, and biotechnology research and development services. List one department for each service area and indicate its contribution to patient care.

	Department	Service Area	Contribution to Patient Care
Example:			
	Nursing	Therapeutic	Treats patient by performing procedures
1.	_____	_____	_____
2.	_____	_____	_____
3.	_____	_____	_____
4.	_____	_____	_____
5.	_____	_____	_____

■ Worksheet 2

Health Occupations and Service Areas

Identify one health occupation in each of the health service areas (diagnostic, therapeutic, informatics, support, and biotechnology research and development). List one duty to illustrate why the occupation falls within this service area.

	Occupation	Service	Duty
Example:			
	Echocardiography Technologist	Diagnostic	Tests to help determine the condition of the heart in order to make a diagnosis
1.	_____	_____	_____
2.	_____	_____	_____
3.	_____	_____	_____
4.	_____	_____	_____
5.	_____	_____	_____

Health Care Tour

Your teacher will help you arrange a tour of a local hospital or another health care organization, individually or working in pairs with a classmate. Choose a specific department, unit, or service that's of interest to you. Tour the area and speak with a representative who works there. Either during or after your tour, complete the answers to the following questions:

1. What department, unit, or service did you choose? What is the function or role of this area?

2. What types of patients do they serve?

3. What types of workers are employed in the area and what are their main duties?

4. What educational requirements are needed to work in the area?

5. Do workers need a license or certification? If so, what are the requirements?

6. What are the advantages of working in this area?

7. What are the challenges of working in this area?

Ask other appropriate questions to find out all you can about this area, and record what you learned in the following space.

After your visit, give a brief oral report to your classmates and teacher.

■ Worksheet 4

Matching Key Terms with Definitions

Key Terms #1: Match each term with its correct definition:

_____ 1. acute

_____ 2. alternative medicine

_____ 3. aseptic

_____ 4. career ladder

_____ 5. career lattice

_____ 6. clerical

_____ 7. chronic

_____ 8. deviation

_____ 9. discharging

_____ 10. dispense

a. to distribute or pass out

b. using healing arts which are not part of traditional medical practice in the United States

c. of or pertaining to keeping records, filing, typing, or other general office tasks

d. occurs frequently over a long period of time

e. departure from a standard or norm

f. a vertical sequence of job positions to increase rank and pay

g. severe but over a short period of time

h. free from the living germs of disease

i. related job positions offering vertical and lateral movement

j. the act of releasing or allowing to leave

k. entering the body

Key Terms #2: Match each term with its correct definition:

_____ 1. entry-level

_____ 2. euthanize

_____ 3. extract

_____ 4. full-time

_____ 5. genes

_____ 6. geriatric

_____ 7. outpatient

_____ 8. invasive

_____ 9. multiskilled

a. a place to receive medical care without being admitted to a hospital; or a person who receives medical care someplace other than a hospital

b. cross-trained to perform more than one function, often in more than one discipline

c. specializing in health care for elderly patients

d. a starting position for someone with little or no experience

e. identify and take out or emphasize

f. entering the body

g. actions taken to avoid a medical condition

h. to painlessly end the life, or permit the death, of a hopelessly sick or injured animal or individual for reasons of mercy

i. working approximately 40 hours per week

j. a portion of DNA that contains instructions for a trait

Key Terms #3: Match each term with its correct definition:

_____ 1. perioperative

_____ 2. portfolio

_____ 3. prenatal

_____ 4. preventive

_____ 5. primary care

_____ 6. specialists

_____ 7. standards

_____ 8. transferable skills

a. three phases of surgery, from the time a decision is made to have surgery, through the operation itself, and until the patient has recovered

b. skills acquired in one job that are applicable in another job

c. accepted basis of comparison in measuring quality or value

d. actions taken to avoid a medical condition

e. basic medical care that a patient receives upon first contact with the health care system, before being referred to specialists

f. people devoted to a particular occupation or branch of study

g. collection of materials that demonstrate knowledge, skills, and abilities

h. a starting position for someone with little or no experience

i. occurring before birth

Chapter 2 • Working in Health Care
Section 2.1 Work Ethic and Performance

■ **Objectives**

After completing this section, you will be able to:

1. Define the key terms.
2. Explain the difference between *soft skills* and *hard skills* and discuss why health care workers need both types of skills.
3. Define *interdependence* and *systems perspective* and explain their importance in health care.
4. Explain why it's important to be "present in the moment" at work.
5. Define *critical thinking* and list three things that critical thinkers do to make good decisions.
6. List five factors that demonstrate a strong work ethic.
7. Describe the attitudinal differences between optimists and pessimists.
8. Discuss the importance of confidentiality, HIPAA, and the HITECH Act.
9. Identify how competence and scope of practice impact quality of care.
10. List two things you should do when representing your employer.
11. Explain the purpose of performance evaluations.
12. Differentiate between objective and subjective evaluation criteria.

■ **Directions**

1. Read Section 2.1 in your textbook.
2. Complete Worksheet 1.
3. Complete Worksheet 2.
4. Complete Worksheet 3.
5. Complete Worksheet 4.
6. Complete Worksheet 5.

■ **Evaluation Method**

- Worksheets
- Class participation
- Section test

Demonstrating a Strong Work Ethic

1. List five factors that demonstrate a strong work ethic. Then list five factors that could lead to dismissal from your job.

Demonstrates a Strong Work Ethic

1. _____

2. _____

3. _____

4. _____

5. _____

Could Lead to Job Dismissal

1. _____

2. _____

3. _____

4. _____

5. _____

Adapting to Change

At a staff meeting this morning, the manager announced that work schedules are changing in order to provide better service to patients. Employees who currently work from 8:00 am to 4:30 pm will need to change their hours to 7:00 am to 3:30 pm. The evening shift will also start one hour earlier, working from 3:30 pm to midnight. In addition to being open on weekdays Monday through Friday, the department will soon begin scheduling patients on Saturdays from 8:00 am to 2:00 pm. Employees who sign-up to work on Saturdays will have Mondays off. A new 10-hour shift is being created for people who would like to work four 10-hour days per week.

In the following space, write a brief paragraph that describes how an optimist might react to these changes.

Write a second paragraph that describes how a pessimist might react to these changes.

Write a third paragraph that describes how *you* might react to these changes if you worked in this facility.

How do think a health care professional would react to these changes? Explain your answer.

Mission, Values, and Reputation

Does your school have a mission statement? If so, locate the mission statement and write it in the following space. If you can't locate a mission statement for your school, write one yourself in the following space. Include your school's "special duties, functions, or purposes."

In the following space, list your school's values, or "beliefs held in high esteem."

Create an organizational chart showing the components of your school and how they fit together. Where do the students fit into this picture?

In the following space, write three examples of ways in which school leaders, teachers, and students must depend on each other to fulfill the school's mission and values.

1.

2.

3.

Compare your work with your classmates' work. Identify similarities and differences. Describe what you and your classmates can do to support the mission, values, and reputation of your school.

Similarities:

Differences:

Things my classmates and I can do:

Problem Solving

In the following space, briefly describe a problem that you faced within the last month. List the steps you took to solve the problem.

Describe the outcome. Did you get the results you wanted or needed? Why, or why not? Explain your answer.

If the steps you took did not solve the problem to your satisfaction, make a new list of steps that might have worked better.

What have you learned from this exercise, and how might you approach problem solving differently in the future?

■ Worksheet 5

Matching Key Terms with Definitions

Key Terms #1: Match each term with its correct definition:

_____ 1. compliance

_____ 2. conflict of interest

_____ 3. constructive criticism

_____ 4. contingency plans

_____ 5. corrective action

_____ 6. discretion

_____ 7. fraud

_____ 8. people skills

_____ 9. impaired

_____ 10. initiative

_____ 11. insubordination

_____ 12. hard skills

_____ 13. cooperation

a. steps taken to overcome a job performance problem

b. offering positive input on another person's weaknesses with the goal of their improvement

c. the ability to perform the technical, hands-on duties of a job

d. refusal to complete an assigned task

e. an inappropriate relationship between personal interests and official responsibilities

f. intentional deceit through false information or misrepresentation

g. backup plans in case the original plans don't work

h. something done on purpose

i. acting in accordance with laws and with a company's rules, policies, and procedures

j. taking the first step or move

k. a reduced ability to function properly

l. being careful about what one says and does

m. personality characteristics that enhance your ability to interact effectively with other people; also known as soft skills

n. acting or working together for a common purpose

Key Terms #2: Match each term with its correct definition:

_____ 1. intentional

_____ 2. objective

_____ 3. peers

_____ 4. rational

_____ 5. reasoning

_____ 6. reliable

_____ 7. responsibility

_____ 8. stagnant

_____ 9. subjective

_____ 10. subordinates

_____ 11. interpersonal skills

_____ 12. soft skills

_____ 13. personality

a. the ability to interact with other people

b. forming conclusions based on coherent and logical thinking

c. a reduced ability to function properly

d. without motion; dull, sluggish

e. based on reason, logical

f. people at a lower rank

g. people at the same rank

h. something done on purpose

i. distinctive individual qualities of a person, relating to patterns of behavior and attitudes

j. a sense of duty binding someone to a course of action

k. affected by a state of mind or feelings

l. can be counted upon; trustworthy

m. personality characteristics that enhance your ability to interact effectively with other people; also known as people skills

n. what is real or actual; not affected by feelings

Key Terms #3: Match each term with its correct definition:

_____ 1. critical thinking

_____ 2. HIPAA

_____ 3. dismissal

_____ 4. job description

_____ 5. front-line workers

_____ 6. employers of choice

_____ 7. HITECH Act

_____ 8. diligent

_____ 9. corporate values

_____ 10. interdependence

_____ 11. hostile workplace

_____ 12. optimists

_____ 13. corporate mission

_____ 14. work ethic

a. special duties, functions, or purposes of a company

b. beliefs held in high esteem by a company

c. using reasoning and evidence to make decisions about what to do or believe without being biased by emotions

d. careful in one's work

e. involuntary termination from a job

f. companies where people like to work

g. employees who have the most frequent contact with a company's customers

h. Health Insurance Portability and Accountability Act of 1996; national standards to protect the privacy of a patient's personal health information

i. Health Information Technology for Economic and Clinical Health Act of 2009; national standards to protect the confidentiality of electronically transmitted patient health information

j. an uncomfortable or unsafe work environment

k. measurement of success in executing job duties

l. attitudes and behaviors that support good work performance

m. the need to rely on one another

n. a document that describes a worker's job duties

o. people who look on the bright side of things

Key Terms #4: Match each term with its correct definition:

_____ 1. punctual

_____ 2. self-awareness

_____ 3. 360 degree feedback

_____ 4. social networking sites

_____ 5. whistle blower

_____ 6. unethical

_____ 7. sexual harassment

_____ 8. systematic

_____ 9. problem solving

_____ 10. systems perspective

_____ 11. reimbursement

_____ 12. up-code

_____ 13. probationary period

_____ 14. pessimists

_____ 15. performance evaluation

_____ 16. organizational chart

a. illustration showing the components of a company and how they fit together

b. people who look on the dark side of things

c. a testing or trial period to meet requirements

d. using a systematic process to solve problems

e. an uncomfortable or unsafe work environment

f. arriving on time

g. to pay back or compensate for money spent

h. understanding where you are, what you're doing, and why you're doing it

i. unwelcome, sexually-oriented advances or comments

j. Internet places for people to publish and share personal information

k. a methodical procedure or plan

l. stepping back to view an entire process to see how each component connects with the others

m. a violation of standards of conduct and moral judgment

n. modifying the classification of a procedure to increase financial reimbursement

o. a person who exposes the illegal or unethical practices of another person or of a company

p. feedback about an employee's job performance that is provided by peers, subordinates, team members, customers, and others who have worked with the employee who is undergoing evaluation

q. measurement of success in executing job duties

Section 2.2 Your Personal Traits and Professional Image

■ Objectives

After completing this section, you will be able to:

1. Define the key terms.
2. Define *character*, *personal values*, and *morals* and explain how they affect your reputation as a professional.
3. List four examples that demonstrate a lack of character in the workplace.
4. Explain how attire, grooming, hygiene, and posture impact a professional image.
5. Describe how grammar and vocabulary affect your professional image.
6. Discuss the importance of maintaining professionalism after hours.
7. Explain the importance of good time management skills and list three time management techniques.
8. Explain the importance of good personal financial management skills and list three financial management techniques.
9. Explain the importance of good stress management skills and list three stress management techniques.
10. Define *adaptive skills* and explain why the ability to manage change is important in health care.

■ Directions

1. Read Section 2.2 in your textbook.
2. Complete Worksheet 1.
3. Complete Worksheet 2.
4. Complete Worksheet 3.
5. Complete Worksheet 4.
6. Complete Worksheet 5.

■ Evaluation Method

- Worksheets
- Class participation
- Section test

Displaying a Professional Image

List five examples of professional and unprofessional attire:

Professional Attire	**Unprofessional Attire**
1. _____	_____
2. _____	_____
3. _____	_____
4. _____	_____
5. _____	_____

List five examples of professional and unprofessional hygiene and grooming:

Professional Hygiene and Grooming	**Unprofessional Hygiene and Grooming**
1. _____	_____
2. _____	_____
3. _____	_____
4. _____	_____
5. _____	_____

In the following space, write a paragraph that explains the purpose of a dress code in the workplace. Explain how attire, grooming, hygiene, and posture affect a person's professional image.

■ **Worksheet 2**

Character Traits

Review the list of character traits that are explained in Section 2.2 of your textbook. In the following space, list the top five character traits, in rank order, that are most important to you when choosing your friends. Indicate why that trait is important to you.

Top five character traits I look for when choosing my friends:

	Character Trait	**Why this trait is important to me**
1.	_____	_____
2.	_____	_____
3.	_____	_____
4.	_____	_____
5.	_____	_____

List the top five character traits, in rank order, that you believe best describe your own character. Indicate why that trait is important to you.

My top five personal character traits:

	Character Trait	**Why this trait is important to me**
1.	_____	_____
2.	_____	_____
3.	_____	_____
4.	_____	_____
5.	_____	_____

Are the traits that you look for in friends the same as, or different from, the traits you chose to describe your own character? Discuss your answer in the following space.

■ Worksheet 3

Time Management

Think about how you spend your time by preparing and maintaining a time journal for seven consecutive days. In a separate notebook, record each of your activities and the amount of time you spent performing them. At the end of the week, review your journal and develop a list of at least five categories into which you can place each activity. For example, categories might include preparing meals and eating, bathing and dressing for school, attending class, studying and doing assignments, watching TV or surfing the Internet, doing volunteer work, spending time with family and friends, and so forth. Write your list of categories in the following space:

	Category	Total Time/Week
#1	_____	_____
#2	_____	_____
#3	_____	_____
#4	_____	_____
#5	_____	_____

Calculate the total amount of time you spent during the week performing the activities within each category, and record the total time in the space above. Is this what you expected, or are you surprised by some of your results? Record your thoughts in the following space.

■ Worksheet 4

Personal Management Skills

Think about how you spend your time (as determined in Worksheet #3) and how you manage your personal finances and your stress. List one goal for each personal management category (time, finances, and stress) that describes an improvement you would like to make, or an outcome you would like to see occur. List one action step you could take to achieve each goal.

Examples: You might extend your study time by one hour on Monday through Thursday to free up Saturday afternoon to volunteer at a local food pantry. You might save all of your pocket change for a month to treat a friend to dinner. Or you might join a study group to reduce your stress when it's time for final exams.

Time Management:

Goal_____ Action Step: _____

Personal Financial Management:

Goal _____ Action Step: _____

Stress Management:

Goal _____ Action Step: _____

■ Worksheet 5

Matching Key Terms with Definitions

Key Terms #1: Match each term with its correct definition:

_____	1. adaptive skills	a.	a person's moral behavior and qualities
_____	2. character	b.	standards for attire and appearance
_____	3. groomed	c.	the ability to adjust to change
_____	4. dress code	d.	comparison of options to decide which is best
_____	5. conscience	e.	clean and neat
_____	6. cheating	f.	the capability of differentiating between right and wrong
_____	7. morals	g.	deceiving by trickery
_____	8. integrity	h.	body cleanliness
_____	9. judgment	i.	moral judgment that prohibits or opposes the violation of a previously recognized ethical principle
_____	10. hygiene	j.	of sound moral principle
_____	11. time management	k.	the total impression created by a person
		l.	the ability to organize and allocate one's time to increase productivity

Key Terms #2: Match each term with its correct definition:

_____	1. personal financial management	a.	the position of the body or parts of the body
		b.	the ability to make sound decisions about personal finances
_____	2. personal skills	c.	the ability to manage time, finances, stress, and change
_____	3. personal values	d.	things of great worth and importance to a person
_____	4. personal image	e.	the total impression created by a person
_____	5. personal management skills	f.	the ability to manage aspects of your life outside of work
		g.	beliefs that are mainly false about a group of people
_____	6. stereotypes	h.	of sound moral principle
_____	7. posture	i.	system of word structures and arrangements
_____	8. procrastinate	j.	the ability to deal with stress and overcome stressful situations
_____	9. trustworthiness	k.	to postpone or delay taking action
_____	10. grammar	l.	ability to have confidence in the honesty, integrity, and reliability of another person
_____	11. stress management		

Section 2.3 Teamwork and Diversity

■ Objectives

After completing this section, you will be able to:

1. Define the key terms.
2. List three ways to strengthen relationships at work.
3. Explain the roles of courtesy, etiquette, and manners in the workplace.
4. Identify two types of workplace teams and give an example of each.
5. Discuss the roles and responsibilities of health care team members.
6. Define *consensus* and explain why it is important, but difficult, to achieve.
7. Explain the value of having a team mission statement and group norms.
8. Explain why health care workers need to be culturally competent.
9. Explain how culture influences behavior.
10. Identify culturally acceptable and effective gestures, terms, and behaviors.
11. Identify common folk medicine practices.
12. Explain how understanding cultural beliefs affects you as a health care worker.

■ Directions

1. Read Section 2.3 in your textbook.
2. Complete Worksheet 1.
3. Complete Worksheet 2.
4. Complete Worksheet 3.
5. Complete Worksheet 4.
6. Complete Worksheet 5.

■ Evaluation Method

- Worksheets
- Class participation
- Section test

Group Dynamics

Think back to a team or a committee on which you recently served. Answer the following questions and give some examples.

1. Did the group work well together? Why or why not?

2. Did the group have a mission statement?

3. Were the team or committee's goals well defined?

4. What roles did the members play?

5. Who took the leadership role? Why did this occur and how did it happen?

6. How well did the members communicate with one another?

7. Were group norms used?

8. How did you feel about the role that you played in the group and your overall experience as a member of it?

9. Were your ideas and opinions respected?

10. How could the team or committee have functioned better?

■ Worksheet 2

Generational Differences

Generational differences can have a huge impact at work. It's important to understand how members of the different generations view their work and their jobs. Awareness of generation-related diversity factors is especially important for health care managers who must recruit, supervise, and retain skilled personnel.

Interview two people who are older than you. One should be a member of the Baby Boomer Generation, born between the 1940s and 1960s. The other person should be a member of Generation X, born between the 1960s and 1980s. The purpose of your interviews is to identify differences (diversity) based upon the era in which people grew up. Discuss the following generational characteristics, and ask the person if he or she feels the description is accurate.

Circle the accurate factors and strike-out the inaccurate factors. Based on information gathered through your interviews, list some additional characteristics for the two generations. Then think about your own generation—Generation Y, born between the 1980s and the year 2000. List some of the characteristics which are unique to your generation.

Baby Boomers:

- Largest generation on earth; result of the post World War II baby boom

- Every life stage has been trend setting; their impact can't be ignored

- Attitude: "If you have it, flaunt it."

- Competitive, stylish, bossy, and curious

- Like shopping, leading, creating a vision

- Dislike paying debts and growing older

- Entered the workforce when the economy was growing; ample jobs after college

- Are staying in their jobs longer; keeping Gen Xers from "moving up the ladder"

- _____

- _____

- _____

Generation X

- Unlike baby boomers, they arrived almost unnoticed

- The economic boom was fading; they watched their parents struggle with employment

- May have been *latch-key kids*; were independent and could figure things out on their own

- The cynical generation; invented the term, "Whatever...."

- Broken homes and divorce were common; may have been raised by one parent or by two sets of parents

- Value friends, relationships, and loyalty
- Caught in the middle of economic change and companies in transition
- Naturally impatient; thrive on change
- They expect to be respected; but it may take time for them to respect other people
- Like surprises, fun, and humor at work
- Dislike being micromanaged
- _____
- _____
- _____

Generation Y

- Arrived when society and the media were focused on babies and children
- Grew up with technology, so it comes naturally to them
- Want to get involved and make the world a better place
- Caring, honest, optimistic, clean-cut
- Like shopping, friends, family, the environment
- Dislike dishonesty and unbalanced lifestyles
- Respond to leaders who show integrity
- Like to be challenged, try new things, and learn in a hands-on manner
- Want to learn continually; expect the workplace to provide growth opportunities
- Work isn't their life; they fit work into life
- Will leave an organization if work/life balance and growth aren't included
- _____
- _____
- _____

List two things that you should do to support teamwork when members of your team are from these generations:

Baby Boomers: _____   _____

Generation X: _____   _____

Generation Y: _____   _____

■ **Worksheet 3**

Culture and Health Care Beliefs

Divide into groups of four to five students per group. Each group should plan to build a health clinic in a community of a different culture. If your school is located in a multicultural community, choose cultures in your town. Develop a presentation (to give to your classmates) to convince the leaders of this community to let you build the clinic. You must research the culture's health care beliefs so you know how to focus your oral presentations to the community leaders.

In the following space, write the name of the culture that you picked and four of the culture's health care beliefs identified through your research.

Culture: _____

Health care beliefs:

1. _____

2. _____

3. _____

4. _____

List two barriers that you might encounter in convincing the community leaders. Explain how you would overcome these barriers:

Potential Barrier	**How to Overcome the Barrier**
1. _____	_____
2. _____	_____

■ Worksheet 4

Cultural Differences

1. Using information from Section 2.3 of your textbook, match the name of each of the following cultures in the space next to the relevant statement. Use only those that apply. Some cultures may be used more than once.

   Cambodian   Anglo-American   Vietnamese
   African-American   Navajo   Japanese
   Southeast Persian   Mexican-American   Laotian

   _____ a. This culture only allows a parent to touch the head of a child.

   _____ b. This culture only allows the elderly to touch the head of a child.

   _____ c. The people of this culture avoid eye contact as a form of respect.

   _____ d. The people of this culture use peripheral vision instead of direct eye contact.

   _____ e. In this culture, people do not shake hands in greeting.

   _____ f. In this culture, people greet one another with a salute.

2. Indicate which of the following cultures is a *close-contact* or *more-distant contact* culture.

   X for close-contact culture   *O* for more-distant culture

   _____ a. Latin American

   _____ b. American

   _____ c. Canadian

   _____ d. Mediterranean

   _____ e. Northern European

   _____ f. African

   _____ g. Southern European

   _____ h. English

   _____ i. Indonesian

■ Worksheet 5

Matching Key Terms with Definitions

Key Terms #1: Match each term with its correct definition:

_____ 1. prejudge

_____ 2. civility

_____ 3. bias

_____ 4. cultural competence

_____ 5. etiquette

_____ 6. polite

_____ 7. delegate

_____ 8. inclusive

_____ 9. diversity

_____ 10. cohesiveness

_____ 11. disparities

_____ 12. body language

a. state of being well integrated or unified

b. to give another person responsibility for doing a specific task

c. acceptable standards of behavior in a polite society

d. to decide or make a decision before having the facts

e. a tendency to include everyone

f. politeness, consideration

g. courteous, having good manners

h. differences, dissimilarities, variations

i. favoring one way over another, based in having had some experience

j. the ability to interact effectively with people from different cultures

k. lack of similarity or equality; health disparities: unfair and misdiagnosis and treatment

l. the power to reach goals and get results

m. nonverbal messages communicated by posture, hand gestures, facial expressions, etc.

Key Terms #2: Match each term with its correct definition:

_____ 1. productivity

_____ 2. role

_____ 3. prohibit

_____ 4. expertise

_____ 5. colleagues

_____ 6. ad hoc

_____ 7. courtesy

_____ 8. golden rule

_____ 9. discipline

_____ 10. facilitator

_____ 11. cliques

_____ 12. loyalty

a. for a specific purpose

b. the power to reach goals and get results

c. to not allow

d. a position, responsibility, or duty

e. polite behavior, gestures, and remarks

f. a branch of knowledge or learning

g. treat other people the way you want to be treated

h. small, exclusive circles of people

i. connections between or among people

j. fellow workers in the same profession

k. high degree of skill or knowledge

l. a person responsible for leading or coordinating a group or discussion

m. showing faith to people that one is under obligation to defend or support

Key Terms #3: Match each term with its correct definition:

_____ 1. long-term goals

_____ 2. conflict

_____ 3. consensus

_____ 4. short-term goals

_____ 5. traditional

_____ 6. manners

_____ 7. interpersonal relationships

_____ 8. interdisciplinary

_____ 9. compromise

_____ 10. mission statement

_____ 11. group norms

_____ 12. synergy

a. a settlement of disagreement between parties by each party agreeing to give up something that it wants

b. a contradiction, fight, or disagreement

c. reaching a decision that all members agree to support

d. expectations or guidelines for group behavior

e. involving two or more disciplines

f. connections between or among people

g. aims that will take a relatively long time to achieve

h. standards of behavior based on thoughtfulness and consideration of other people

i. a summary describing aims, values, and an overall plan

j. aims that will take a relatively short time to achieve

k. people working together in a cooperative action

l. customary beliefs passed from generation to generation

m. a position, responsibility, or duty

Chapter 3 • Communication in Health Care

Section 3.1 Interpersonal Communication

■ **Objectives**

After completing this section, you will be able to:

1. Define the key terms.
2. Explain why communication is important.
3. Name four elements that may influence how you communicate with others.
4. List three barriers to communication.
5. List four elements necessary for communication to take place.
6. Describe three things that a good listener does.
7. Differentiate between verbal and nonverbal communication.
8. Describe the four styles of communication, and explain why assertive communication works best.
9. Discuss the importance of conflict resolution skills.
10. Explain the importance of anger management.
11. Describe the role that defense mechanisms play.

■ **Directions**

1. Read Section 3.1 in your textbook.
2. Complete Worksheet 1.
3. Complete Worksheet 2.
4. Complete Worksheet 3.
5. Complete Worksheet 4.
6. Complete Worksheet 5.

■ **Evaluation Method**

- Worksheets
- Class participation
- Section test

Sending and Receiving Messages

For this activity, you will work in groups of two. Choose a partner and sit back-to-back. You will each have an identical set of colored squares, circles, triangles, and so on. One of you will be the *sender* of messages and one of you will be the *receiver*.

The sender will put the colored pieces down one by one to create a design, without the receiver being able to see it. The sender will describe his or her design clearly enough so that the receiver can make an exact replica of it. Only the sender may speak; the receiver may not ask questions.

When the receiver has replicated the sender's design, stop and compare the two designs.

- Are the designs alike, or are they different? Why?
- How well did the communication go between the sender and the receiver?
- Were the sender's directions exact and clear?
- What could have been done to make the communication better?

Change roles and repeat the activity.

Once you have both had a turn as a sender and a receiver, reflect on this communication activity. How did this activity help you:

- Discover that words mean different things to different people?
- Identify words that indicate clear directions?
- Appreciate the value of two-way communication where both people send and receive messages and provide feedback?

In the following space, describe what you learned from this activity that could help improve your interpersonal communication skills.

■ Worksheet 2

The Four Styles of Communication

Consider each of the following scenarios and decide which style of communication each scenario demonstrates. Insert your answer using: AS for *assertive*; AG for *aggressive*; P for *passive*; or PA for *passive-aggressive.*

Scenario #1

Becky has just returned to her work area after disappearing for 30 minutes without telling anyone where she was going or why she was leaving. Her coworker says:

_____ "It's about time you showed up. Where have you been? I'm getting fed up with you just disappearing all the time and leaving me to do our work!"

_____ "There you are. I finished our work for the afternoon."

_____ "There you are. I finished our work for the afternoon." (You don't know it yet, but I'm going to disappear on you for an entire hour tomorrow morning when we're swamped and have a deadline to meet. Let's see how *you* like working alone!)

_____ "I'm concerned there's so much paperwork to complete and it's a two-person job. Is there something I can help you with to get us back to work on meeting this deadline? "

Scenario #2

Lawrence and Joann are serving on a committee to revise their clinic's dress code. The leader of the group asks for suggestions. Joann wants to establish *casual day* on Fridays so she can wear blue jeans and sports jerseys. Lawrence works at the public reception desk and feels that casual dress presents an unprofessional image for his organization. When Joann brings up the topic of casual Fridays, Lawrence responds:

_____ "If that's what you want, it's okay with me." (Our dress code says no blue jeans or sports jerseys, so there's no way our manager will approve this. I'll make sure he knows this was Joann's crazy idea.)

_____ "Dressing casually one day a week would be fun and something to look forward to. But would casual attire comply with our dress code standards for a professional environment?"

_____ "You've got to be kidding me! There's no way that blue jeans are allowed in our corporate dress code no matter what day of the week it is. Do you have any other stupid ideas?"

_____ "If you want a casual day, I guess it's okay with me."

Compare answers with your classmates and discuss any disagreements.

In the following space, write a brief description of what might happen when people use aggressive, passive, or passive-aggressive communication styles. What might happen when people use the assertive style? Which style is most effective, and why?

■ Worksheet 3

Symbolic Language

Do some research to learn how vision impaired people communicate using Braille and how hearing impaired people communicate using sign language. Also research the use of interpreters.

In the following space, write a paragraph about each form of communication to describe how it originated and how it works.

Braille:

Sign language:

Locate some examples of Braille and sign language and exchange them with your classmates. Learn five basic phrases in sign language and practice using them to communicate with your classmates. List the five phrases here:

1.

2.

3.

4.

5.

In the following space, describe how health care workers could use Braille and sign language to communicate with their blind and deaf patients.

Write a brief statement to explain how the family members and friends of blind or deaf patients might help overcome communication barriers with health care workers.

Write a brief statement to describe the role of interpreters and explain how interpreters help overcome communication barriers in health care.

When You Were Confronted

Recall a time when someone confronted you, and you had to deal with interpersonal conflict. Perhaps the person accused you of some wrong doing or felt that you didn't do something you were supposed to do. Maybe the person thought you took something of theirs or disrespected their feelings or opinions. Perhaps the person voiced criticism of your work or felt you were guilty of inappropriate behavior.
In the following space, describe the confrontation. Include:

- What caused the conflict?

- Who was involved?

- Why did the person confront you?

- How, when, and where did the confrontation take place?

- What style of communication did the person use, and why?

- How did you react, and why?

- How did the conversation go?

- What happened as a result?

- Was the conflict resolved? Why or why not?

- Could things have been handled differently or better? If so, explain how.

- What did you learn from the experience?

- What, if anything, do you think the other person might have learned from the experience?

When You Confronted Someone

Now, recall a time when *you* confronted another person. In the following space, describe the confrontation. Include:

- What caused the conflict?

- Who was involved?

- Why did you confront the person?

- How, when, and where did the confrontation take place?

- What style of communication did you use, and why?

- How did the other person react, and why?

- How did the conversation go?

- What happened as a result?

- Was the conflict resolved? Why or why not?

- Could you have handled things differently or better? If so, explain how.

- What did you learn from the experience?

- What, if anything, do you think the other person might have learned from the experience?

- How might this experience affect how you confront people and handle conflict in the future?

- What resources could you have used to help ensure the confrontation did not escalate?

When You Became Angry

Recall the last time you became angry because of something that someone said or did to you. In the following space, describe the situation. Include:

- What caused your anger?

- What happened and who was involved?

- What communication took place?

- How did you feel about the situation?

- How did you respond?

- Were other people affected? If so, how?

- What influence, if any, did the person's words or actions have on your behavior?

- Did the person *press your buttons* and cause you to react in a certain way?

- Did the person have control over your behavior? Why or why not?

- Was your anger resolved? Why or why not?

- Could you have handled things differently or better? If so, explain how.

- What did you learn from the experience?

- How might this experience affect how you handle your anger in the future?

- What resources could you have used to help ensure the situation did not escalate?

■ Worksheet 5

Matching Key Terms with Definitions

Key Terms #1: Match each term with its correct definition:

_____ 1. assertive

_____ 2. impatience

_____ 3. passive

_____ 4. confrontation

_____ 5. engagement

_____ 6. passive-aggressive

_____ 7. aggressive

_____ 8. annoyance

a. behavior aimed at causing harm or pain

b. irritation

c. bold, confident, self-assured

d. to face boldly, defiantly, or antagonistically

e. securing the attention of a person

f. restlessness

g. accepting or allowing an action without response

h. appearing passive, but aggressive in behavior

i. describing a person with a word that limits them

Key Terms #2: Match each term with its correct definition:

_____ 1. conflict resolution

_____ 2. workplace bullies

_____ 3. labeling

_____ 4. dialect

_____ 5. inferior

_____ 6. defense mechanisms

_____ 7. slang

a. lower or less than

b. describing a person with a word that limits them

c. overcoming disagreements between two or more people

d. the informal language of a particular group

e. employees who intimidate and belittle their coworkers

f. mental devices that help people cope with various situations

g. a variety of language that is distinct to a culture

h. irritation

Section 3.2 Electronic Communication and Computers in Health Care

■ Objectives

After completing this section, you will be able to:

1. Define the key terms.
2. List key factors in the appropriate use of telephones, fax machines, e-mail, and the Internet at work.
3. Describe *texting* and explain why texting abbreviations should not be used at work.
4. List five potential mistakes when communicating electronically and explain how to prevent them.
5. Explain why computer security at work is important and list two ways to protect computer security.
6. Describe the roles of web browsers, Internet search engines, and domain names.
7. Describe the basic components and functions of computers.
8. List two examples of how computers are used in therapeutic and diagnostic services.
9. Discuss computer security issues related to the use of laptops, PDAs and flash drives.
10. Explain why people need computer skills to work in health care.

■ Directions

1. Read Section 3.2 in your textbook.
2. Complete Worksheet 1.
3. Complete Worksheet 2.
4. Complete Worksheet 3.
5. Complete Worksheet 4.
6. Complete Worksheet 5.

■ Evaluation Method

- Worksheets
- Class participation
- Section test

■ Worksheet 1

Advantages, Disadvantages, and Risks

Think about the advantages, disadvantages, and risks of using electronic communication and computers in health care. In the following space, list the advantages, disadvantages, and risks from the viewpoint of the patients, workers, and health care organizations. Do the advantages outweigh the disadvantages and risks? Write a brief paragraph to explain your answer.

1. **Advantages of Electronic Communication and Computers in Health Care**

   For patients:

   For workers:

   For health care organizations:

2. **Disadvantages of Electronic Communication and Computers in Health Care**

   For patients:

   For workers:

   For health care organizations:

3. **Risks of Using Electronic Communication and Computers in Health Care**

For patients:

For workers:

For health care organizations:

4. **Do the advantages outweigh the disadvantages and risks in certain cases? Why or why not?**

■ Worksheet 2

E-mail Communication

Write an e-mail memorandum to be sent to ten health care workers who are employed by several different hospitals around your state. The memo is an invitation to participate in a half-day conference one month from now to discuss emergency preparedness. The conference agenda covers four topics, including the need to update the state's five-year-old plan for responding to natural disasters such as floods and tornados. Your e-mail memorandum should not only invite guests to the conference but also provide them with the agenda and a copy of the state's current plan.

Write your e-mail memo in the following space. Then list the steps you will take to send the information and to make certain that each of the invited guests is planning to participate.

■ Worksheet 3

Text Messaging Abbreviations

Compile a list of commonly used text messaging abbreviations by doing some online research and speaking with your classmates, family members, and friends. Using the e-mail memorandum that you wrote for Worksheet #2 above, rewrite your memorandum in the following space using several text messaging abbreviations in place of complete words.

Show your memorandum to someone who is not familiar with text messaging. Ask the person to read your message and explain its purpose and content. You may need to ask the person some questions to determine if he or she clearly understood the communication. In the following space, write a brief paragraph discussing the issues that might arise when health care workers use text messaging abbreviations in their communication at work.

■ Worksheet 4

Communicating with Patients

Each of the following questions is inappropriate when speaking with a patient in person or by telephone. Rewrite each question in the space provided to make the question more appropriate.

1. What's your name? _____

2. What did you say? _____

3. Can't you speak up? _____

4. Don't you speak English? _____

5. Can't you hear very well? _____

6. What do you want? _____

7. Huh? _____

List five key factors in providing good customer service when communicating with people in person or by telephone:

1.

2.

3.

4.

5.

■ Worksheet 5

Matching Key Terms with Definitions

Key Terms #1: Match each term with its correct definition:

_____ 1. blind carbon copy

_____ 2. first responders

_____ 3. emoticons

_____ 4. attachment

_____ 5. apps

_____ 6. recipient

_____ 7. cover page

_____ 8. carbon copy

_____ 9. memorandum

_____ 10. facsimile or fax machine

a. software applications for smartphones and computerized hand-held devices

b. a file linked to an e-mail message

c. an e-mail feature that allows a person to send an e-mail to multiple people without them seeing the other receivers' e-mail addresses

d. an e-mail feature that allows a person to send a copy of an e-mail to another person

e. the first page of a fax or a written report

f. use of punctuation marks and letters in an e-mail message to convey the sender's emotions

g. to produce information; turn out

h. a short note written to help a person remember something, or to remind a person to do something

i. a person or thing that receives

j. a device that sends and receives printed pages or images as electronic signals over telephone lines

k. the first people to appear and take action in emergency situations

Key Terms #2: Match each term with its correct definition:

_____ 1. electronic health records

_____ 2. Internet search engines

_____ 3. intranet

_____ 4. output

_____ 5. password

_____ 6. Internet

_____ 7. flash drive

_____ 8. domain name

_____ 9. input

_____ 10. central processing unit

a. the part of a computer that interprets and carries out instructions

b. the Internet address for a web page

c. medical records kept via computer

d. a small memory device used to store and transport files among computers; also known as a thumb drive or jump drive

e. to enter data into a computer for processing

f. the worldwide computer network with information on many subjects

g. programs that search documents for keywords and produce lists where the keywords were found

h. a private computer network with limited access

i. to produce information; turn out

j. a secret series of numbers and letters that identifies the person who should have access to a computer, file, or program

k. a person or thing that receives

Key Terms #3: Match each term with its correct definition:

_____ 1. homeostasis

_____ 2. telerobotics

_____ 3. data mining

_____ 4. HEDIS

_____ 5. transparency

_____ 6. comparative data

_____ 7. tomography

_____ 8. mortality rate

a. information gathered from multiple sources that is analyzed to identify similarities and differences

b. sifting through large amounts of data to find significant information

c. an organization that provides quality care guidelines

d. constant balance within the body

e. a file linked to an e-mail message

f. the ratio of deaths in an area to the population of that area, over a one-year period

g. open, clear, and capable of being seen

h. robots controlled from a distance using wireless connections

i. radiographic technique that produces a scan showing detailed cross-sections of tissue

Key Terms #4: Match each term with its correct definition:

_____ 1. telemedicine

_____ 2. smartphones

_____ 3. username

_____ 4. personal digital assistant

_____ 5. Web browser

_____ 6. website

_____ 7. tweets

_____ 8. texting

a. a small, mobile, hand-held computerized device

b. mobile telephones that have advanced computing and connectivity features

c. the use of telecommunications technology to provide patient care in remote areas where patients and caregivers cannot meet in person

d. sending real-time, short text messages between cell phones or other handheld devices; also known as text messaging

e. text-based messages of up to 140 characters

f. a unique identifier composed of letters and numbers used as a means of initial identification to gain access to a computer system or Internet service provider

g. a software application that allows users to locate and access Internet web pages

h. a group of pages on the Internet developed by a person or organization about a topic

i. robots controlled from a distance using wireless connections

Section 3.3 Health Information Technology and Communication

■ Objectives

After completing this section, you will be able to:

1. Define the key terms.
2. List two functions and two benefits of health information technology.
3. List the four types of information contained in patient records.
4. Differentiate between subjective and objective observations.
5. List two advantages and two disadvantages of electronic health records.
6. Explain the roles of root word, prefix, and suffix in medical terminology.
7. Describe why correct spelling is so important when using medical terms.
8. List four elements of effective written communication.
9. Explain the benefit of using charts, graphs, and tables in written documents.
10. List four elements of effective oral presentations.

■ Directions

1. Read Section 3.3 in your textbook.
2. Complete Worksheet 1.
3. Complete Worksheet 2.
4. Complete Worksheet 3.
5. Complete Worksheet 4.
6. Complete Worksheet 5.

■ Evaluation Method

- Worksheets
- Class participation
- Section test

■ Worksheet 1

Electronic Health Records

Think about the advantages, disadvantages, and risks of using electronic health records instead of paper health records. In the following space, list the advantages, disadvantages, and risks from the viewpoint of the patients, workers, and health care organizations.

Advantages of Electronic Health Records

For patients:

For workers:

For health care organizations:

Disadvantages of Electronic Health Records

For patients:

For workers:

For health care organizations:

Risks of Using Electronic Health Records

For patients:

For workers:

For health care organizations:

Do the advantages outweigh the disadvantages and risks in all cases? Write a brief paragraph to explain your answer.

■ Worksheet 2

Observations and Patient Health Records

1. List four senses you would use for making observations about patients:

   a. _____

   b. _____

   c. _____

   d. _____

2. In the following space, explain the difference between subjective and objective observations by giving the definition of each term and listing two examples:

   Subjective observations:

   Definition _____

   Example 1 _____

   Example 2 _____

   Objective observations:

   Definition _____

   Example 1 _____

   Example 2 _____

3. List six examples of information that must be included in all patient health records:

   a. _____

   b. _____

   c. _____

   d. _____

   e. _____

   f. _____

Proofreading and Making Corrections

Proofread the following memorandum. Circle improper language, spelling, grammar, and punctuation. Then rewrite the document in the following space to incorporate your corrections. Make sure your memo provides clear and complete information and reflects the elements of effective written communication.

Date: March 22, 2012

Subject: March 21 Workshop on Records

To: All Employes

Our workshop on Electronic Health Record will take place on March 20 from ten to 4. Will meet in room 210 in the ambultory care center. Bring lunch if you want too. Pete from Info Tech will due the training and explain how this effects us. His assistant and him will do checkoffs afterward. If you wasn't at the last meeting, it don't matter. Will have the notes for you. UR must arrive on time and stay 4 the hole time. We will take a break @ noon. See you then.

■ Worksheet 4

Written and Oral Communication

List six elements of effective written communication:

1.

2.

3.

4.

5.

6.

Describe three things that might happen if a business document does not meet the standards for effective written communication:

1.

2.

3.

List six elements of effective oral presentations:

1.

2.

3.

4.

5.

6.

Describe three things that might happen if a presentation at work does not meet the standards for effective oral presentations:

1.

2.

3.

■ Worksheet 5

Matching Key Terms with Definitions

Key Terms #1: Match each term with its correct definition:

_____	1. executive summary	a.	the main part of a letter or other written document
_____	2. documentation	b.	to write observations or records of patient care
_____	3. font	c.	the primary reason why a patient seeks medical care
_____	4. legible	d.	the ending portion of letter
_____	5. closing	e.	limited to persons authorized to use information or documents
_____	6. chart	f.	expressed in few words
_____	7. body	g.	greeting
_____	8. confidential	h.	a record of something
_____	9. concise	i.	a brief overview listing the major points of a business document
_____	10. chief complaint	j.	style of type
		k.	hand-writing that can be read and accurately interpreted by another person

Key Terms #2: Match each term with its correct definition:

_____	1. salutation	a.	professional stationery imprinted with business contact information
_____	2. spell check	b.	graphic image that represents a company or organization
_____	3. logo	c.	something that is noted
_____	4. proofread	d.	expressed in few words
_____	5. subject line	e.	reference containing information on medical diseases, conditions, and drugs
_____	6. PDR	f.	reviewing a document for errors
_____	7. observations	g.	greeting
_____	8. thesaurus	h.	software that verifies the correct spelling of words
_____	9. standard of care	i.	the type of care that would be reasonably expected under similar situations
_____	10. letterhead	j.	a statement describing the subject of a letter
		k.	reference source for locating alternate words with similar meanings

Chapter 4 • The Health Care Industry
Section 4.1 The History of Health Care

■ Objectives

After completing this section, you will be able to:

1. Define the key terms.
2. Identify three scientists and explain what they contributed to medicine.
3. Choose one era in the history of health care and explain how medical knowledge and technology changed during that time.
4. Describe the role of Florence Nightingale in advancing the role of nursing.
5. List two trends that led to the emergence of the allied health professions.
6. Give two examples of allied health professions.
7. Name two advances in medicine in the twentieth century.
8. Identify a possible advancement in medicine for the twenty-first century.
9. List two ethical questions or problems resulting from medical advancements.

■ Directions

1. Read Section 4.1 in your textbook.
2. Complete Worksheet 1.
3. Complete Worksheet 2.
4. Complete Worksheet 3.
5. Complete Worksheet 4.
6. Complete Worksheet 5.

■ Evaluation Method

- Worksheets
- Class participation
- Section test

■ Worksheet 1

The Hippocratic Oath

Research the modern version of the Hippocratic Oath and select one of the statements. In the following space, write a brief paragraph discussing: 1) how the statement applies in medicine today, and 2) how the statement applies to all health care workers, not just physicians.

Designing a Research Project

Design an imaginary research project using the scientific method to solve a problem. The problem can be something involving your work, your classes at school, or your personal life. Use these six steps in your design:

1. State a problem or ask a question.

2. Gather background information.

3. Form a hypothesis.

4. Design and perform an experiment.

5. Draw a conclusion.

6. Report the results.

In the following space, state your problem or ask your question. Make a list of the steps you would take to gather background information. Form your hypothesis and write it down. Record the steps you would take to design and perform your experiment. Imagine that you implemented your experiment. Then write your conclusions based on what you think would happen and report your results.

1. My problem/question:

2. The steps I would take to gather background information:

3. My hypothesis:

4. The steps I would take to design and perform my experiment:

5. My conclusions based on what I think would happen:

6. My results:

In the following space, answer the following questions:

1. What did you learn from this experience?

2. What might happen if you actually implemented your experiment?

Scientists and Their Contributions to Medicine

Identify nine scientists, and explain what they contributed to medicine.

1. _____

2. _____

3. _____

4. _____

5. _____

6. _____

7. _____

8. _____

9. _____

■ Worksheet 4

Current Medical Research

Bring an article from a newspaper, magazine, medical journal, or the Internet to class that describes one example of current medical research. In the space below, answer the following questions:

1. What is the purpose of the research?

2. Who is conducting the research, and where is it occurring?

3. What is the researchers' hypothesis?

4. What type of experiment is being conducted?

5. What do the researchers hope to learn from their work?

6. If the research is successful, who will benefit from it?

■ Worksheet 5

Matching Key Terms with Definitions

Key Terms #1: Match each term with its correct definition:

_____ 1. anatomy

_____ 2. antiseptic

_____ 3. baseline data

_____ 4. accurate

_____ 5. benchmark

_____ 6. continuous quality improvement

_____ 7. anesthesia

_____ 8. adverse effects

_____ 9. custodial

_____ 10. best practice

_____ 11. convents

a. exact, correct, or precise

b. unfavorable or harmful outcomes

c. the science of dealing with the structure of animals and plants

d. loss of feeling or sensation

e. substance that slows or stops the growth of microorganisms

f. gathering information before a change begins to better understand the current situation

g. information gathered after a change has occurred to examine the impact or results

h. a standard by which something can be measured or compared

i. a method or technique that has consistently shown superior results through research and experience as compared with other methods and techniques

j. the regular use of methods and tools to identify, prevent, and reduce the impact of process failures

k. establishments of nuns

l. marked by watching and protecting rather than seeking to cure

Key Terms #2: Match each term with its correct definition:

_____ 1. intravenously

_____ 2. metrics

_____ 3. microorganisms

_____ 4. midwives

_____ 5. life expectancy

_____ 6. epidemics

_____ 7. microbiology

_____ 8. exorcise

_____ 9. hypothesis

_____ 10. dissection

a. not involving penetration of the skin

b. act or process of dividing, taking apart

c. diseases affecting many people at the same time

d. to force out evil spirits

e. an explanation for an observation that is based on scientific research and can be tested

f. directly into a vein

g. the number of years of life remaining at any given age

h. a set of measurements that quantify results

i. the branch of biology dealing with the structure, function, uses, and modes of existence of microscopic organisms

j. organisms so small that they can only be seen through a microscope

k. non-physician women who deliver babies

Key Terms #3: Match each term with its correct definition:

_____ 1. monasteries

_____ 2. outcome data

_____ 3. phlebotomy

_____ 4. psychiatry

_____ 5. noninvasive

_____ 6. process

_____ 7. physiology

_____ 8. primitive

_____ 9. predators

_____ 10. pasteurization

_____ 11. pathogens

a. homes for men following religious standards

b. not involving penetration of the skin

c. a set of measurements that quantify results

d. information gathered after a change has occurred to examine the impact or results

e. microorganisms or viruses that can cause disease

f. to heat food for a period of time to destroy certain microorganisms

g. the practice of opening a vein by incision or puncture to remove blood

h. the branch of biology dealing with the functions and activities of living organisms and their parts

i. organisms or beings that destroy

j. ancient or prehistoric

k. set of actions or steps that must be accomplished correctly and in the proper order

l. the practice or science of diagnosing and treating mental disorders

Key Terms #4: Match each term with its correct definition:

_____ 1. psychology

_____ 2. respiration

_____ 3. root cause

_____ 4. symptoms

_____ 5. readmission

_____ 6. superstitious

_____ 7. vaccine

_____ 8. stethoscope

_____ 9. replicate

_____ 10. quackery

_____ 11. Six Sigma

a. the science of the mind or mental states and processes

b. the practice of pretending to cure disease

c. a quick return to the hospital after discharge

d. to reproduce or make an exact copy

e. the inhaling and exhaling of air, or breathing

f. the factor that, when fixed, will solve a problem and prevent it from happening again

g. a strategy that uses data and statistical analysis to measure and improve an organization's operational performance

h. an instrument used to hear sound in the body, such as heartbeat, lung sounds and bowel sounds

i. ancient or prehistoric

j. trusting in magic or chance

k. a sign or indication of something

l. a weakened bacteria or virus given to a person to build immunity against a disease

Section 4.2 Health Care Today

■ Objectives

After completing this section, you will be able to:

1. Define the key terms.
2. List five types of health care facilities and describe their roles.
3. List four government agencies involved in health care and describe their roles.
4. Explain how not-for-profit organizations provide support for health care, and list two examples.
5. Discuss the difference between the service side and the business side of health care.
6. List three reasons for the rising cost of health care.
7. Describe the impact on patients and health care providers when people don't have health insurance or a family doctor.
8. Explain the concept of managed care and how it is different from fee-for-service.
9. Give three examples of how providers have modified their practices to provide quality health care at a lower cost.
10. Describe three types of health insurance organizations and programs.
11. Explain the purpose of HEDIS.
12. Discuss health care reform efforts, including two strategies and two issues of concern.

■ Directions

1. Read Section 4.2 in your textbook.

2. Complete Worksheet 1.

3. Complete Worksheet 2.

4. Complete Worksheet 3.

5. Complete Worksheet 4.

6. Complete Worksheet 5.

■ Evaluation Method

- Worksheets
- Class participation
- Section test

■ Worksheet 1

Hospital Departments

In the following space, list five departments found in a general hospital. For each department, answer the following questions: What is the main purpose of the department? What is one health care service that the department provides?

Example: Dietetics department; main purpose is to provide food for patients, workers, and visitors; provides nutrition for patients based on their dietary treatment plans.

Department #1

Department #2

Department #3

Department #4

Department #5

■ Worksheet 2

Health Care Facilities and Agencies

In the following space, list five different kinds of health care facilities or agencies and identify the purpose of each.

Example: Nursing homes provide residences for people who require constant nursing care and have significant problems with activities of daily living.

Facility/Agency #1

Facility/Agency #2

Facility/Agency #3

Facility/Agency #4

Facility/Agency #5

■ Worksheet 3

The Rising Cost of Health Care

List three reasons why the cost of health care is so expensive today:

1.

2.

3.

List three strategies currently being used to reduce the cost of health care, and briefly explain how each strategy works:

1.

2.

3.

List three strategies under debate that might reduce the cost of health care in the future, and briefly explain how each strategy might work:

1.

2.

3.

In the following space, write a brief paragraph describing what *you* think should be done to reduce the cost of health care.

List three things that *you* can do as a consumer of health care to reduce the cost of health care services:

1.

2.

3.

■ **Worksheet 4**

The Baby Boomers' Demand for Health Care Services

List six things that need to happen in the next ten years in order to meet the baby boomers' increasing demand for health care services:

1.

2.

3.

4.

5.

6.

■ Worksheet 5

Matching Key Terms with Definitions

Key Terms #1: Match each term with its correct definition:

_____ 1. accountability

_____ 2. bulk

_____ 3. chiropractic

_____ 4. communicable

_____ 5. constant

_____ 6. compensation

_____ 7. ambulatory

_____ 8. benefits

_____ 9. co-insurance

_____ 10. audiology

_____ 11. accountable care organizations

_____ 12. complementary medicine

a. willing to accept responsibility and the consequences of one's actions

b. networks where hospitals and doctors work together and share accountability to manage all of the health care needs of a large group of Medicare patients for an extended period of time

c. able to walk

d. the study of hearing disorders

e. payments and assistance based on an agreement

f. continuous, connected, and coordinated

g. a greater amount

h. the method of adjusting the segments of the spinal column

i. a percentage the subscriber is required to pay of every medical bill

j. capable of being passed directly or indirectly from one person or thing to another

k. payment

l. combining alternative medical approaches with traditional medical practices

m. fixed, unchanging

Key Terms #2: Match each term with its correct definition:

_____ 1. defensive medicine
_____ 2. eligibility
_____ 3. endowments
_____ 4. consumers
_____ 5. facilities
_____ 6. continuity
_____ 7. gatekeepers
_____ 8. environmental sanitation
_____ 9. co-payment
_____ 10. deductible
_____ 11. convalescence

a. the periodic payment to Medicare, an insurance company, or a health care plan for health care or prescription drug coverage

b. people who purchase or use a product or service

c. continuous, connected and coordinated

d. the gradual recovery of health and strength after illness

e. a set amount the subscriber pays for each medical service

f. an amount the subscriber must pay before the insurance begins to pay

g. medical practices aimed at avoiding lawsuits rather than benefitting the patient

h. the quality or state of being qualified

i. gifts of property or money given to a group or an organization

j. methods used to keep the environment clean and to promote health

k. places designed or built to serve a special function; such as a hospital, clinic, or doctor's office

l. people who monitor the actions of other people and who control access to something

Key Terms #3: Match each term with its correct definition:

_____ 1. hydrotherapy
_____ 2. legislation
_____ 3. gross domestic product
_____ 4. malpractice
_____ 5. intervention
_____ 6. managed care
_____ 7. maternal
_____ 8. hypertension
_____ 9. infant mortality rate
_____ 10. immunizations
_____ 11. health care exchanges

a. GDP; the total market value of all good and services produced in one year

b. open marketplaces where buyers and sellers of health insurance come together to help consumers compare and shop for coverage

c. organizations that deliver primary care through a comprehensive team approach that ensures quality outcomes

d. treatment that uses water therapy for disease or injury

e. elevation of the blood pressure

f. substances given to make disease organisms harmless to the patient; may be given orally or by injection, such as for tetanus and polio

g. the number of infants that die during the first year of life

h. the act of interfering to change an outcome

i. a law or body of laws

j. negligence, failure to meet the standard of care or conduct pre-scribed by a profession

k. a health care system where primary care doctors act as gatekeepers to manage each patient's care in a cost-effective manner

l. relating to the mother or from the mother

Key Terms #4: Match each term with its correct definition:

_____ 1. Medicare

_____ 2. Medicaid

_____ 3. orthopedics

_____ 4. perspective

_____ 5. premium

_____ 6. podiatry

_____ 7. mobility

_____ 8. occupational therapy

_____ 9. obstetrics

_____ 10. obese

_____ 11. medical homes

a. a government program that provides health care for low-income people and families and for people with certain disabilities

b. organizations that deliver primary care through a comprehensive team approach that ensures quality outcomes

c. a set amount the subscriber pays for each medical service

d. a government program that provides health care primarily for people 65 and older

e. the ability to move from place to place without restriction

f. weighing more than 20% over a person's ideal weight

g. the branch of medical science concerned with childbirth

h. helps to give people skills for everyday activities in order to lead satisfying lives

i. the medical specialty concerned with correcting problems with the skeletal system

j. the manner in which a person views something

k. the diagnosis and treatment of foot disorders

l. the periodic payment to Medicare, an insurance company, or a health care plan for health care or prescription drug coverage

Key Terms #5: Match each term with its correct definition:

_____ 1. rehabilitation

_____ 2. specialties

_____ 3. system

_____ 4. trends

_____ 5. refer

_____ 6. recreational therapy

_____ 7. urology

_____ 8. stakeholders

_____ 9. prosthetics

_____ 10. surgical

a. artificial parts made for the body, such as teeth, feet, legs, arms, hands, eyes, breasts

b. the manner in which a person views something

c. uses play, recreation, and leisure activities to improve physical, cognitive, social, and emotional functioning; the primary goal is to develop lifetime leisure skills

d. to send to

e. process that helps people who have been disabled by sickness or injury to recover as many of their original abilities for activities of daily living as possible

f. fields of study or professional work, such as pediatrics, orthopedics, obstetrics

g. people with a keen interest in a project or organization; may be end-users of a product or service

h. repairing or removing a body part by cutting

i. a coordinated body of methods or plans of procedure

j. general direction or movement

k. the study of the urine and urinary organs in health and disease

Chapter 5 • Finding the Right Occupation for You

Section 5.1 Career Planning and Self-Discovery

■ **Objectives**

After completing this section, you will be able to:

1. Define the key terms.
2. Explain the role that dreaming plays in career planning.
3. Describe the importance of having a career plan and a vision statement.
4. List the characteristics of SMART goals and explain why goals are necessary.
5. Discuss the role that self-discovery plays in career planning.
6. List three types of career assessments and explain their value.
7. Discuss how identifying your motivations, values, personality type, and interests can help you select a career that matches your needs and preferences.
8. List three skills included in the Framework for 21st Century Learning.
9. Discuss the importance of identifying your knowledge, skills, and abilities when considering career options.

■ **Directions**

1. Read Section 5.1 in your textbook.
2. Complete Worksheet 1.
3. Complete Worksheet 2.
4. Complete Worksheet 3.
5. Complete Worksheet 4.
6. Complete Worksheet 5.

■ **Evaluation Method**

- Worksheets
- Class participation
- Section test

■ Worksheet 1

The Milestones in My Life

Think about the important *milestones* in your life, things that have happened that made a significant impact on you. In the following space, list at least ten of these milestones and the approximate date they occurred, starting with your birth date. Use extra paper if necessary. Here's an example:

- Born February 5, 1997
- Started first grade, September 2002
- Won Little League baseball tournament, June 2005
- Started babysitting, April 2009
- Awarded a blue ribbon at the county fair, August 2010
- Won 2nd place in the Science Fair, March 2011
- Got my first job, April 2012
- Earned Perfect Attendance award at school, June 2012
- Elected vice president of my high school class, October 2012
- Got my driver's license, July 2013

Previous Milestones in my Life:

✔ _____

✔ _____

✔ _____

✔ _____

✔ _____

✔ _____

✔ _____

✔ _____

✔ _____

✔ _____

What milestones do you anticipate in your future? In the following space, continue your list. Use extra paper if necessary. Start with completing your high school education or obtaining your GED, and then think ahead about what might occur as you mature and become self-dependent. Include milestones such as enrolling in college or a training program, starting your first health care job, getting married, starting a family, excelling in a favorite sport or hobby, and so forth. Try to come up with at least ten future milestones and their approximate dates. As mentioned in your textbook, it's time to do some dreaming.

Anticipated Milestones in my Future:

✔ _____

✔ _____

✔ _____

✔ _____

✔ _____

✔ _____

✔ _____

✔ _____

✔ _____

✔ _____

In the following space, write a brief paragraph discussing how this exercise can help you with career planning.

■ Worksheet 2

My Vision Statement and Motivations

An important part of career planning is having a dream or a vision for your future. Review the section in your textbook titled, "Writing Your Vision Statement." In the following space, write a brief paragraph that describes what you want your future to look like. Focus on the role that your job and career will play in your life. Think about your priorities and include them in your vision statement.

My vision statement:

Knowing and understanding what motivates you is another key aspect of career planning. Review the section in your textbook titled, "Finding Out What Motivates You." In the following space, list three things that motivate you now and three things that you think will motivate you as you launch your career plan.

Things that motivate me now:

1. _____

2. _____

3. _____

Things that I think will motivate me as I launch my career plan:

1. _____

2. _____

3. _____

In the following space, write a brief paragraph that describes what you think will motivate you if the *going gets rough* in achieving your career goals.

My Personal Values and Work Values

Another element in career planning is identifying your personal values and your work values. What things do you value the most? Review the section in your textbook titled, "Identifying Your Values." From the list of twenty-five personal values, choose the ten that are most important to you. In the following space, list your ten personal values in rank order, with value #1 being the most important.

My personal values:

1. _____

2. _____

3. _____

4. _____

5. _____

6. _____

7. _____

8. _____

9. _____

10. _____

Review the section in your textbook titled, "The More You Know: Work Values and Careers." From the list of six work values, choose the three that are most important to you. In the following space, list your three work values in rank order, with value #1 being the most important.

My work values:

1. _____

2. _____

3. _____

In the following space, write a brief paragraph that describes the role your personal and work values will play in choosing your health career.

Matching My Personality Type and Interests to Health Careers

Step 1. The occupation you choose should be a good match for your personality type and your individual preferences. Review the material in Section 5.1 in your textbook titled, "Learning About Your Personality Type."

Step 2. If your teacher is using the textbook's companion website for your course, complete the Golden Personality Type Profiler assessment. If you don't have access to this assessment, proceed to the next step.

Step 3. Review "John Holland's Interest Theory" in Section 5.1 in your textbook. Read the descriptions for each of the personality types, and use the information to identify which three types sound most like you.

Write your three-letter Holland code here: _____

Step 4. If possible, take Holland's Self-Directed Search assessment online to help you identify your interests as well as your skills. This assessment requires a small fee. Go to http://www.self-directed-search.com/. The report will identify your 3-letter Holland code. You can then use your code to match careers using O*Net Online.

Step 5. Now it's time to match your personality type and interests to different health careers. Based on your 3-letter Holland code, use the O*NET Online (www.onetonline.org) *Advanced Search* to find at least ten health careers that match your type. List the ten careers below, and circle the five careers that sound most interesting to you:

1. _____

2. _____

3. _____

4. _____

5. _____

6. _____

7. _____

8. _____

9. _____

10. _____

Step 6. In the following space, write a brief paragraph that discusses what you've learned from this exercise. Were there any surprises? How can you use this information to research careers? Do the careers that you've listed align with your motivations and values?

■ Worksheet 5

Matching Key Terms with Definitions

Key Terms #1: Match each term with its correct definition:

_____ 1. abilities   a. people who focus on the outer world

_____ 2. capabilities   b. fundamental aptitudes in reading, language, and math

_____ 3. assessments   c. motivated by external influences

_____ 4. basic skills   d. flexible work schedule with no guaranteed hours or benefits

_____ 5. extrinsic   e. things that draw the attention of a person

_____ 6. extroverts   f. motivated by internal influences

_____ 7. intrinsic   g. goals that are specific, measurable, attainable, relevant and time bound

_____ 8. interests   h. a vivid and idealized picture of the future

_____ 9. motivations   i. underlying enduring traits useful in performing tasks

_____ 10. SMART goals   j. potential abilities

_____ 11. supplemental   k. tools or processes to gather information

_____ 12. vision statement l. forces that move you to set goals and achieve them

_____ 13. career plan   m. people who focus on their inner world

                                n. strategy for a person's professional growth and development

Key Terms #2: Match each term with its correct definition:

_____ 1. occupation   a. important elements in a person's life

_____ 2. preferences   b. people who focus on their inner world

_____ 3. part-time   c. things that stand in the way or oppose progress

_____ 4. introverts   d. a person's job to earn a living

_____ 5. prestigious   e. working approximately 20 hours a week

_____ 6. secondary   f. giving priority or advantage to some things over other things

_____ 7. skills   g. admired and respected, of high esteem

_____ 8. recognition   h. receiving credit for achievement

_____ 9. vision   i. high school

_____ 10. values   j. potential abilities

_____ 11. self-discovery   k. the process of learning about one's self

_____ 12. obstacles   l. capabilities that can be acquired and developed through a learning, practice, and repetition

_____ 13. work values   m. a mental image to imagine what the future could be

                                n. global aspects of work that are important to a person's satisfaction

Section 5.2 Career Exploration and Preparation

■ Objectives

After completing this section, you will be able to:

1. Define the key terms.
2. Identify three resources for career exploration.
3. Describe the value of role models and mentors.
4. List five key questions to ask when conducting occupational research.
5. Explain the role that labor trends and projections play in career exploration.
6. List four key questions to ask when choosing a school.
7. List four key questions to ask when choosing an educational program.
8. Describe the criteria that selection committees use to make admission decisions for schools.
9. Describe the criteria that selection committees use to make admission decisions for educational programs.
10. Name three types of funding and financial aid to help pay educational expenses.
11. List five things you should do in high school to prepare for your health career.

■ Directions

1. Read Section 5.2 in your textbook.
2. Complete Worksheet 1.
3. Complete Worksheets 2A, 2B, and 2C.
4. Complete Worksheet 3.
5. Complete Worksheet 4.
6. Complete Worksheet 5.

■ Evaluation Method

- Worksheets
- Class participation
- Section test

■ Worksheet 1

My Accomplishments

One way to gain confidence in taking that first big step in your career is to focus on things that you've already accomplished in your life. Recognizing your accomplishments also helps you identify your knowledge, skills, and abilities (KSAs). Your accomplishments reflect where you've been, what you've achieved, and what you're capable of doing in the future. Accomplishments are evidence of your strengths and your skills.

In the following space, list the top five major accomplishments in your life. Refer to *Worksheet 1: The Milestones in My Life* in the previous section of this *Student Activity Guide* to jog your memory. This information will be helpful when you draft your résumé and complete applications for school and for financial aid and jobs.

My Accomplishments:

1. _____

2. _____

3. _____

4. _____

5. _____

In the following space, write a brief paragraph describing how you will use your past accomplishments to gain the confidence and courage you need to develop your potential.

My Career Exploration

Using the *career exploration resources* listed in Section 5.2 of your textbook, answer the following *career exploration questions* for your three top health career choices. Use extra sheets of paper if needed.

Health Career Choice #1 _____

1. What job tasks are required?

2. What knowledge, skills, and abilities are required?

3. What are the education and training requirements?

4. What are the licensing, certification, and/or registration requirements?

5. How much does the job pay?

6. What are the continuing education requirements?

7. What are the opportunities for career advancement and professional development?

8. What are the labor trends and projections for this occupation?

9. Which assessment results led you to consider this career, and why?

■ Worksheet 2B

My Career Exploration

Using the *career exploration resources* listed in Section 5.2 of your textbook, answer the following *career exploration questions* for your three top health career choices. Use extra sheets of paper if needed.

Health Career Choice #2 _____

1. What job tasks are required?

2. What knowledge, skills, and abilities are required?

3. What are the education and training requirements?

4. What are the licensing, certification, and/or registration requirements?

5. How much does the job pay?

6. What are the continuing education requirements?

7. What are the opportunities for career advancement and professional development?

8. What are the labor trends and projections for this occupation?

9. Which assessment results led you to consider this career, and why?

My Career Exploration

Using the *career exploration resources* listed in Section 5.2 of your textbook, answer the following *career exploration questions* for your three top health career choices. Use extra sheets of paper if needed.

Health Career Choice #3 _____

1. What job tasks are required?

2. What knowledge, skills, and abilities are required?

3. What are the education and training requirements?

4. What are the licensing, certification, and/or registration requirements?

5. How much does the job pay?

6. What are the continuing education requirements?

7. What are the opportunities for career advancement and professional development?

8. What are the labor trends and projections for this occupation?

9. Which assessment results led you to consider this career, and why?

■ Worksheet 3

My School and Educational Program Exploration

Select one of the three health career choices you identified in Worksheet 2. Use career exploration resources and resource people to identify an area school and an educational program that prepare students for this career. Answer the following exploration questions. Use extra sheets of paper if needed.

Health Career _____

School Name _____

Program Name _____

School Exploration

1. What is the school's accreditation status?

2. What is the school's reputation?

3. Does the school grant college degrees or certificates of completion?

4. What does the school require for admission?

5. How diverse is the school's student population?

6. What is the average class size?

7. What is the travel distance to the school from your home?

8. Does the schedule of classes offer flexibility?

9. How much does the school cost, and does it offer financial aid?

Educational Program Exploration

1. What is the educational program's accreditation status?

2. What is the educational program's reputation?

3. Does completion of the educational program lead to a college degree or a certificate of completion?

4. What does the educational program require for admission?

5. How diverse is the educational program's student population?

6. What is the average class size?

7. How does the program handle clinical experience?

8. How long is the program and what is the graduation rate?

9. What is the pass rate on board exams for program graduates?

10. What is the job placement and job retention rate for program graduates?

In the following space, write a brief paragraph to describe the extent to which this school and educational program might meet your needs. Explain your answer.

■ Worksheet 4

My SMART Goals

In the space below, write your SMART goals for the health career you have chosen. Include the long- and short-term goals you will need to accomplish along the way. Make sure your goals are specific, measurable, attainable, relevant, and time bound. Here's an example:

My goal is to earn a bachelor's degree in nursing by May 2018 and pass the nursing board exam by the end of that summer. To accomplish this goal, I will:

1. Research local colleges with nursing programs and choose a school by September, 2013.

2. Apply to college by February 2014 and get accepted by June, 2014.

3. Graduate from high school in May, 2014.

4. Start the C.N.A. program at the local Adult Education Center in June, 2014, and complete the program by the end of August.

5. Find a C.N.A. weekend job for 12-15 hours per week by the time college classes start.

6. Start taking college prerequisite courses in English, math, social studies, foreign language, and science (2 semesters) in September, 2014.

7. Apply to the college's nursing program in March, 2015.

8. If not accepted, continue taking courses at the college and improve my grades.

9. If necessary, reapply to the nursing program in March, 2016.

10. Take nursing courses and participate in clinical experiences.

11. In my third year of nursing school, secure a Student Nurse Externship position for the summer in a local hospital.

12. Complete my bachelor's degree in nursing by May 2018.

13. Study for my nursing boards and pass the exam by the end of August, 2018.

My SMART Goals:

What delays, obstacles, or barriers might you face? List five examples and describe what you will do to get back on track if this happens to you:

Delay, Obstacle, or Barrier

1. _____
2. _____
3. _____
4. _____
5. _____

How I Will Get Back on Track

1. _____
2. _____
3. _____
4. _____
5. _____

List five people who could serve as your network of supporters:

1. _____
2. _____
3. _____
4. _____
5. _____

■ Worksheet 5

Matching Key Terms with Definitions

Key Terms #1: Match each term with its correct definition:

_____ 1. formal	a. high school courses that qualify for college credit
_____ 2. advanced placement	b. things that obstruct or impede
	c. based on facts and logical conclusions
_____ 3. intuitive	d. additional instruction for adults who have completed their formal education
_____ 4. HOSA	
_____ 5. job outlook	e. acquiring knowledge and information
_____ 6. job shadowing	f. structured, in accordance with accepted forms and regulations
_____ 7. education	g. grade point average; a measure of a student's academic achievement in school
_____ 8. cognitive	h. the student organization for health occupation students at the secondary, postsecondary, adult, and college level
_____ 9. GPA	
_____ 10. institutional accreditation	i. a quality assurance process to ensure that a school meets high quality standards
	j. the method in which a student learns best
_____ 11. programmatic accreditation	k. a quality assurance process to ensure that an educational program meets high quality standards
_____ 12. continuing education	l. based on instinct and feeling
	m. the demand of a career in a certain field
_____ 13. barriers	n. spending time observing a professional in his or her work environment to see what a typical day is like
_____ 14. drug screen	
_____ 15. felony	o. lab test to detect illegal substances in a job applicant
	p. a major offense with extensive jail time as a penalty

Key Terms #2: Match each term with its correct definition:

_____ 1. labor projections

_____ 2. labor trends

_____ 3. role model

_____ 4. prerequisites

_____ 5. tasks

_____ 6. remedial

_____ 7. rigors

_____ 8. training

_____ 9. learning style

_____ 10. novice

_____ 11. program

_____ 12. projections

_____ 13. mentor

_____ 14. criminal history background check

_____ 15. misdemeanor

a. estimates of the number of positions needed in the future based on labor trends

b. forces that impact employers, workers, and those seeking work

c. based on instinct and feeling

d. the method in which a student learns best

e. a wise, loyal adviser

f. someone new in a field or activity, a beginner

g. required or necessary as a prior condition

h. a planned set of courses and activities to prepare students for a particular career

i. estimates of the number of positions needed in the future

j. correcting a deficiency

k. things that are hard or severe

l. a person whom someone aspires to be like

m. pieces of work, or functions to be performed, as part of a job

n. building skills

o. a review of legal records to search for misdemeanors and felonies

p. a minor offense with a fine and/or short jail sentence as a penalty

Chapter 6 • Working with Patients
Section 6.1 Meeting Patient Needs

■ **Objectives**

After completing this section, you will be able to:

1. Define the key terms.
2. List the three causes of physical disabilities.
3. List three categories of mental illness.
4. Describe one risk factor for mental illness.
5. Name four psychological needs that must be met, and give one example of each need.
6. Name four physiological needs that must be met, and give one example of each need.
7. Describe the five psychological stages that terminally ill patients experience.
8. List three ways to meet the needs of terminally ill patients.
9. Identify two mistakes or errors that jeopardize patient safety.
10. List three ways to protect patient safety.

■ **Directions**

1. Read Section 6.1 in your textbook.
2. Complete Worksheet 1.
3. Complete Worksheet 2.
4. Complete Worksheet 3.
5. Complete Worksheet 4.
6. Complete Worksheet 5.

■ **Evaluation Method**

- Worksheets
- Class participation
- Section test

■ Worksheet 1

Meeting Needs and Restoring Health

A 25-year-old man suffered a head injury from a motorcycle accident which left him partially paralyzed and unable to speak. His daily care provides a bath, clean clothes, and food. People around him rarely speak to him. He stays in his room and looks out the window most of the time.

In the following space, write a paragraph that compares his day with yours. Make specific recommendations that could assist in moving this person toward health as described by the World Health Organization. Explain how your recommendations would help meet this man's needs and improve his health status.

■ Worksheet 2

Meeting the Needs of Terminally Ill Patients

Create a scenario in which you are a terminally ill patient with approximately one month to live.

1. In the following space, write a paragraph that describes:

   - Your medical condition (such as breast or prostate cancer, dementia, renal failure, and so on).

   - When and how your medical condition was diagnosed.

   - Your current state of mind, using Dr. Kübler-Ross' stages of grief.

   - Your current physical condition (pain and discomfort, physical impairments, limitations, and so on).

   - Your ability/disability in performing activities of daily living.

2. List your physiological and psychological needs. Explain what health care workers would need to do to help meet your needs.

3. Describe how you might approach hospice care and what you would want and need from family members and friends. How would you want to be treated? How could family and friends help meet your physiological and psychological needs?

4. List your top five priorities for the final month of your life, and discuss why they are important to you:

5. Discuss what you have learned from this experience that you could apply to your future work as a health care professional.

■ Worksheet 3

National Patient Safety Goals

Locate the current National Patient Safety Goals at www.jointcommission.org/ standards. In the following space, list four of the goals and explain how each goal would improve patient safety:

1.

2.

3.

4.

Write a brief paragraph that explains how increased patient safety would affect the overall function of the health care facility.

Meeting Patient Needs

Consider each of the following medical conditions. Place a DI next to each *debilitating illness*, a MI next to each *mental illness*, and a CC next to each *congenital condition*.

_____ autism

_____ epilepsy

_____ depression

_____ diabetes

_____ attention deficit hyperactivity disorder (ADHD)

_____ leukemia

_____ cerebral palsy

_____ anorexia nervosa

_____ cleft lip

_____ post-traumatic stress disorder (PTSD)

_____ multiple sclerosis (MS)

_____ hydrocephaly

_____ Parkinson's disease

_____ cystic fibrosis

_____ panic attacks

_____ cardiovascular disease

_____ bipolar disorder

_____ Down syndrome

_____ emphysema

_____ schizophrenia

_____ sickle-cell anemia

_____ cancer

_____ drug abuse

_____ alcoholism

_____ AIDS

_____ spinal bifida

Select one of the medical conditions listed on the previous page and write it here:

_____

List three basic human needs that patients who have this condition should have met:

1. _____

2. _____

3. _____

Worksheet 5

Matching Key Terms with Definitions

Key Terms #1: Match each term with its correct definition:

_____ 1. amputation	a. removal of a body part
_____ 2. congenital	b. to shrink and become weak
_____ 3. impending	c. capable of understanding
_____ 4. coherent	d. deep sleep, unconscious state for a period of time
_____ 5. empowered	e. existing at, or before, birth
_____ 6. atrophy	f. causing weakness or impairment
_____ 7. intellectual stimulation	g. something a person is unable to do well due to a mental or physical impairment
_____ 8. elimination	h. process of expelling or removing, especially waste products from the human body
_____ 9. social services	i. to give authority, to enable or permit
_____ 10. staffing level	j. about to happen
_____ 11. disability	k. causing deep thought
_____ 12. debilitating	l. activities and resources to support well-being for individuals and families
_____ 13. coma	m. the number of people with certain qualifications who are assigned to work at a given time
	n. to cause an activity or heightened action

Key Terms #2: Match each term with its correct definition:

_____ 1. mistake

_____ 2. dose

_____ 3. stimulate

_____ 4. isolated

_____ 5. justice

_____ 6. heredity

_____ 7. genetics

_____ 8. error

_____ 9. mental illness

_____ 10. paralysis

_____ 11. holistic

_____ 12. sentinel event

_____ 13. quarantine

a. health condition that changes a person's thoughts, emotions, and behavior and affects that person's ability to undertake daily functions

b. to understand, interpret, or estimate incorrectly

c. loss of sensation and muscle function

d. causing weakness or impairment

e. the quantity of a medicine or a drug that is administered at one time

f. to cause an activity or heightened action

g. an unexpected occurrence involving death or serious physical or psychological injury, or the risk thereof

h. isolating a person or animal to prevent the spread of disease

i. separated, lack of contact with others

j. fairness; applying good rules equally to all people

k. something done incorrectly through ignorance or carelessness

l. traits passed from parent to child through heredity

m. passed from parent to child

n. pertaining to the whole; considering all factors

Section 6.2 Customer Service and Patient Satisfaction

■ Objectives

After completing this section, you will be able to:

1. Define the key terms.
2. List three types of health care customers.
3. Discuss the purpose of patient centered care and list three benefits for patients.
4. Explain the difference between *empathy* and *sympathy*.
5. Describe how hospitals are measuring patient satisfaction.
6. Discuss the purpose of the HCAHPS survey and explain how it is administered.
7. List three concerns that patients may have when they become hospitalized.
8. Explain four ways to provide good customer service for patients.
9. List three ways to provide good customer service for the patient's family members.
10. Describe two ways to provide good customer service for visitors in your facility.

■ Directions

1. Read Section 6.2 in your textbook.
2. Complete Worksheet 1.
3. Complete Worksheet 2.
4. Complete Worksheet 3.
5. Complete Worksheet 4.
6. Complete Worksheet 5.

■ Evaluation Method

- Worksheets
- Class participation
- Section test

Customer Service Experiences

Work in teams of three to four students. Each team will identify at least five examples of poor customer service you have experienced within the last six months. These examples could come from experiences in stores, restaurants, repair shops, online companies, and so forth. Record each example and indicate what should have been done to provide better service.

Examples of Poor Customer Service

1. _____
2. _____
3. _____
4. _____
5. _____

Ways to Improve Customer Service

1. _____
2. _____
3. _____
4. _____
5. _____

What you will do as a result of these poor customer service experiences? Will you return to these places of business again? Why, or why not? Record your answers in the following space.

■ Worksheet 2

Customer Service in Health Care

Think back to your last experience with a health care provider. This could be a family doctor or specialist, a dentist, an eye doctor, a school nurse, a wellness specialist giving free health screenings, and so forth. In the following space, record some examples of the customer service you experienced. Include examples of good customer service and any poor service you might have experienced. Indicate how the poor service should be improved.

Examples of Good Customer Service

_____
_____
_____
_____

Examples of Poor Customer Service

_____
_____
_____
_____

Ways to Improve Customer Service

_____
_____
_____
_____

Based on this experience, are you a satisfied patient? Explain your answer.

Would you recommend this provider to other people? Explain your answer.

Customer Service Scenarios

For each of the following scenarios, describe what you could do as a health care worker to provide excellent customer service for the patient and his or her family and friends. Consider what it would take to *go the extra mile* in each situation. Write your response under each scenario.

Scenario #1

A 20-year-old woman is injured in a car accident on the way to her wedding rehearsal. The wedding is in two days. The bride-to-be will be hospitalized for at least one week with serious, but not life-threatening injuries. Her wedding dress, which was hanging behind the driver's seat, has blood stains but is still wearable. The groom is in the National Guard and scheduled for deployment to Afghanistan within 30 days. The bride and grooms' families, who live more than 1,000 miles away, have arrived in town for the wedding and must return home within three days.

Scenario #2

An 80-year-old man is admitted into a skilled nursing unit after suffering a heart attack and receiving treatment at a nearby hospital. His recovery will take at least one month, and he has no one at home to care for him. With no family or close friends, the man spends most of his time alone. He mentioned that he served overseas in the U.S. Army, and he loves animals, growing houseplants, and doing crossword puzzles.

Scenario #3

A 45-year-old woman comes into the hematology center on a regular basis for chemotherapy to treat her breast cancer. She relies on transportation provided by members of her church, and it's obvious that she has very limited resources. Her chemotherapy treatments take several hours, and she has read all of the magazines provided for the center's patients. She mentioned that she likes mystery novels and biographies, but you know she can't afford to buy them. She used to knit and crochet, but the supplies are too expensive.

■ Worksheet 4

Patient Satisfaction Scores Online

Do some Internet research to see how hospitals are posting the results of their patient satisfaction surveys online for public viewing. Go to the Hospital Compare website at www.hospitalcompare.hhs.gov.

In the *Location* box, enter your zip code, city, or state. Under *Search Type*, choose *General*, *Medical Conditions*, or *Surgical Procedures*. Then click on *Find Hospitals*. Choose three hospitals and click on *Compare*.

Review the comparative statistics for *Survey of Patients' Hospital Experiences*. Click on *View Graphs* and *View Tables* to see how your three hospitals compare with national and state averages.

Using the left navigation, review comparative statistics for *Process of Care Measures* and *Outcome of Care Measures* for your three hospitals.

Using the following space, fill in the information requested.

1. List three of the quality measures which are reported in the *Survey of Patients' Hospital Experiences* section. (Example: Patients who reported that their nurses always communicated well.)

   1. _____

   2. _____

   3. _____

2. List three of the quality measures which are reported in the *Process of Care Measures* section. (Example: Outpatients who are having surgery who got an antibiotic at the right time—within one hour before surgery; higher numbers are better.)

   1. _____

   2. _____

   3. _____

3. List three of the quality measures which are reported in the *Outcome of Care Measures* section. (Example: Death rate for heart attack patients.)

1. _____

2. _____

3. _____

4. List two other types of helpful information that you can find on this website:

1. _____

2. _____

5. Describe how the information on this website can be helpful to patients.

6. Describe how the information on this website could help, or hurt, the reputation of a hospital.

7. Explain how this website provides *transparency* among health care providers.

■ Worksheet 5

Matching Key Terms with Definitions

Key Terms #1: Match each term with its correct definition:

_____ 1. engaged

_____ 2. indifferent

_____ 3. judgmental

_____ 4. amenities

_____ 5. divulge

_____ 6. dictate

_____ 7. remarkable

_____ 8. clergy

a. pleasant and attractive features or benefits

b. people who perform religious functions

c. maintaining the privacy of certain matters

d. record patient information for medical records

e. unusual, uncommon, and extraordinary

f. to make known

g. involved

h. showing no interest or concern

i. having or expressing a critical point of view

Key Terms #2: Match each term with its correct definition:

_____ 1. over-the-counter drugs

_____ 2. empathy

_____ 3. H-CAPS/ HCAHPS

_____ 4. inoculation

_____ 5. sympathy

_____ 6. healing environments

_____ 7. false hope

a. understanding and relating to another person's emotions or situation

b. looking forward to something that probably won't happen

c. Hospital Consumer Assessment of Healthcare Providers and Systems

d. physical spaces designed to reduce stress, ensure safety, and uplift the spirits of patients, visitors, and staff

e. to introduce an antibody or antigen to prevent a disease

f. medications and supplements that don't require a prescription

g. feeling sorrow or pity for another person

h. maintaining the privacy of certain matters

Chapter 7 • Your Legal and Ethical Responsibilities
Section 7.1 Legal Responsibilities

■ **Objectives**

After completing this section, you will be able to:

1. Define the key terms.
2. Describe the rights to which a patient is entitled.
3. List the patient's responsibilities in the health care process.
4. Explain what might happen if health care workers fail to meet their legal responsibilities.
5. Define *licensure, certification,* and *registration,* and explain the role they play.
6. Summarize the importance of patient confidentiality.
7. Explain the purposes of HIPAA and the HITECH Act.
8. Describe the elements of a contract.
9. List the types of advance directives and explain their purpose.
10. Identify the difference between civil law and criminal law.
11. List six common categories of medical malpractice.

■ **Directions**

1. Read Section 7.1 in your textbook.
2. Complete Worksheet 1.
3. Complete Worksheet 2.
4. Complete Worksheet 3.
5. Complete Worksheet 4.
6. Complete Worksheet 5.

■ **Evaluation Method**

- Worksheets
- Class participation
- Section test

■ Worksheet 1

Making Health Care Decisions

In the following space, write a scenario describing a patient who needs a health care proxy decision maker. Include a description of the patient's condition, why he or she can't make his or her own medical decisions, and some examples of the types of decisions that would need to be made on the patient's behalf. List the criteria that the patient should use when choosing his or her proxy.

In the following space, write another scenario where *you* are a patient who is unable to make your own health care decisions. Make a list of what you would, and would not, want your proxy to decide on your behalf. What criteria would you use in choosing your proxy? Explain your answer.

Medical Malpractice

Consider each of the following situations. Decide if the provider has committed medical malpractice or not. Briefly explain your answers.

1. A patient sees his family doctor, complaining of a swollen ankle after playing a game of soccer. He is misdiagnosed. The result is a long term leg injury which later requires surgery.

2. A surgeon is operating on a patient's liver. During the operation, the patient dies of a heart attack. The patient had a very advanced case of heart disease, but the surgeon was unaware of the problem.

3. A nursing home aide is caring for a woman who is 95 years old and in reasonably good health. While the aide is bathing the patient, the patient has a heart attack and dies.

4. A patient with cancer refused chemotherapy and died three months sooner than her physician had expected.

■ Worksheet 3

Scope of Practice

The scope of practice for a health care occupation is usually determined by a state board. Select a health care occupation and research your state's legal scope of practice for that occupation. Summarize your findings in the following space.

List three examples of how a worker in this profession could be found guilty of negligence for violating his or her scope of practice.

1. _____

2. _____

3. _____

Transferring Medical Records

A patient has moved to a different state and has requested that her medical records be transferred from her current primary care doctor to her new doctor. In the space below, create two scenarios. In scenario #1, the confidentiality of her medical records would be protected. In scenario #2, the confidentiality of her medical records would be breached. For each scenario, discuss who was involved, what actions they took (or did not take), and the result. Also discuss the role of HIPAA and the HITECH Act.

Scenario #1

Scenario #2

■ Worksheet 5

Matching Key Terms with Definitions

Key Terms #1: Match each term with its correct definition:

_____ 1. advocates

_____ 2. contract

_____ 3. consent

_____ 4. civil law

_____ 5. criminal law

_____ 6. emancipated

_____ 7. durable power of attorney

_____ 8. advance directive

_____ 9. directive

_____ 10. defamatory

_____ 11. boilerplate language

_____ 12. agent

a. a written instruction such as a living will or a durable power of attorney recognized under state law relating to the provision of health care when the individual is incapacitated

b. people or groups who speak or write in support of something or someone

c. a person or business authorized to act on another's behalf

d. standard language used repeatedly without change

e. the body of law governing certain relationships between people, such as marriage, contracts, and torts

f. approve, agree

g. a legally binding exchange of promises or an agreement between parties that the law will enforce

h. the body of law that defines criminal offenses, deals with the apprehension, charging, and trial of suspected persons, and fixes penalties applicable to convicted offenders

i. statement that causes injury to another person's reputation

j. something that serves to guide or impel towards an action or goal

k. a type of advance medical directive in which legal documents provide the power of attorney, or the authorization to act on someone else's behalf in a legal or business matter, to another person in the case of an incapacitating medical condition

l. legally considered an adult

m. giving approval through an action

Key Terms #2: Match each term with its correct definition:

_____ 1. gross misconduct

_____ 2. incapacitated

_____ 3. legal disability

_____ 4. implied consent

_____ 5. living will

_____ 6. expressed consent

_____ 7. implied contracts

_____ 8. liable

_____ 9. law

_____ 10. expressed contracts

_____ 11. minor

_____ 12. exempt

a. failure to perform in a reasonably prudent manner

b. to be free or released from some liability or requirement to which others are subject

c. giving approval verbally or in writing

d. contracts in which terms are written out in the document

e. unacceptable behavior of a serious nature, often leading to job dismissal

f. permanently or temporarily impaired due to a mental and/or physical condition

g. giving approval through an action

h. contracts in which some terms are not specifically stated, but are understood by the parties based on the nature of the transaction

i. a rule of conduct or procedure recognized by a community as binding or enforceable by authority

j. a person has a disability for legal purposes if he or she has a physical or mental impairment which has a substantial and long-term adverse effect on his or her ability to carry out normal day-to-day activities

k. legally responsible

l. a will in which the signer requests not to be kept alive by medical life-support systems in the event of a terminal illness

m. under the legal age of full responsibility

Key Terms #3: Match each term with its correct definition:

_____ 1. notarized

_____ 2. proxy decision maker

_____ 3. prudent

_____ 4. obligation

_____ 5. registration

_____ 6. principal

_____ 7. misrepresentations

_____ 8. negligence

_____ 9. ombudsman

_____ 10. surrogate

_____ 11. torts

a. untruths, lies

b. failure to perform in a reasonably prudent manner

c. certified as to the validity of a signature

d. legally responsible

e. moral responsibility

f. a social worker, nurse, or trained volunteer who ensures that patients/residents are properly cared for and respected

g. first, or among the first, in importance or rank

h. the advocate for a patient who isn't competent to make decisions about his or her own medical care

i. careful or cautious

j. a list of individuals on an official record who meet the qualifications for an occupation

k. substitute

l. under civil law, wrongs committed by one person against another

Section 7.2 Ethical Responsibilities

■ Objectives

After completing this section, you will be able to:

1. Define the key terms.
2. Explain the difference between unethical and illegal behavior.
3. Identify two factors that influence a person's perspective on right versus wrong.
4. Summarize the code of ethics that every health care worker must follow.
5. List three questions to answer when making ethical decisions.
6. Explain the importance of reporting illegal and unethical conduct.
7. Give two examples of reportable incidences.
8. Identify three resources to help you report illegal or unethical behavior.
9. Identify four examples of complex, controversial bioethical issues.

■ Directions

1. Read Section 7.2 in your textbook.
2. Complete Worksheet 1.
3. Complete Worksheet 2.
4. Complete Worksheet 3.
5. Complete Worksheet 4.
6. Complete Worksheet 5.

■ Evaluation Method

- Worksheets
- Class participation
- Section test

■ Worksheet 1

Ethical Dilemmas

1. You overhear a purchasing agent where you work speaking on the telephone with a salesperson from a local computer company. She offers to buy fifteen new computers for your organization if the salesperson will also agree to sell her son a computer at the same quantity discount.

   In the following space, write a brief paragraph that describes how you would handle this situation. Would you ignore it, or report it? Is the purchasing agent guilty of unethical, illegal, or immoral conduct? Explain your answer.

2. Create an ethical dilemma involving health care organizations, patients, and/ or health care workers. In the following space, describe the dilemma, list options for how to handle the dilemma, and discuss which option you believe would be best.

■ Worksheet 2

Patient Rights

Review the material in Section 7.2 in your textbook that discusses patient rights and select one of them. In the following space, write a brief paragraph describing how the unethical conduct of a health care worker could violate this particular patient right.

Select another patient right. In the space below, write a brief paragraph describing how the illegal conduct of a health care worker could violate this patient right.

Falsifying Data

You are a research assistant working in your local hospital's medical research department. The research involves clinical trials for a new drug to treat cancer patients. Your salary is funded by a grant from the federal government. If the results from the research study are positive, the grant and your job will be renewed for two more years. If the results from the research study are negative or otherwise show no benefit to patients, the project will end in thirty days. One week before the final report is due, the research director tells you to change some of the data to indicate better results.

How would you handle this situation? In the following space, identify your options and explain what you would do. Are there any ethical, legal, or moral issues involved? Could someone be harmed? Would the research director's code of ethics be called into question? Would the hospital's Institutional Review Board (IRB) be involved? Explain your answers.

■ Worksheet 4

Organ Procurement and Transplantation

You serve on a national board to regulate organ procurement and transplantation for hospitals throughout the United States. Consider the ethical, legal, and moral issues surrounding organ transplants. In the following space, record and explain your answers to each of the following questions.

1. Should people be allowed to sell their organs (such as a kidney) to the highest bidder without government interference?

2. What criteria should be used to determine which patients get priority for organ transplants? Consider factors such as age, gender, occupation, medical condition, socioeconomic status, and so on.

3. Should a severely ill, 60-year-old patient who has been a life-long cigarette smoker get a lung transplant before a 45-year-old moderately ill patient who never smoked?

4. Should a wealthy U.S. Senator with ample health insurance have priority for a kidney transplant over a poor and homeless person with no health insurance?

■ Worksheet 5

Matching Key Terms with Definitions

Key Terms #1: Match each term with its correct definition:

_____ 1. appropriate

_____ 2. bioethics

_____ 3. conduct

_____ 4. embryos

_____ 5. dilemma

_____ 6. adverse

_____ 7. code of ethics

_____ 8. clone

_____ 9. clinical trials

_____ 10. anonymous

a. to oppose

b. not named or identified

c. suitable, correct

d. not satisfied by the same set of values

e. ethical decisions that are related to life issues

f. research to evaluate the effectiveness and safety of a medical procedure, device, or drug

g. a group of cells that is genetically identical to the unit from which it was derived

h. principles of conduct for decision making and behavior

i. standard of behavior

j. a difficult situation or problem that requires making a choice

k. living human beings during the first eight weeks of development in the uterus

Key Terms #2: Match each term with its correct definition:

_____ 1. harass

_____ 2. hotline

_____ 3. moral convictions

_____ 4. impartial

_____ 5. reportable incident

_____ 6. project

_____ 7. unbiased

_____ 8. rationed

_____ 9. inconsistent

a. to behave in an offensively annoying or manipulative way

b. standard of behavior

c. direct and immediate telephone assistance

d. not favoring one side or opinion over another

e. not satisfied by the same set of values

f. strong and absolute beliefs about what is right or wrong

g. to show or reflect

h. a fixed portion or amount

i. any event that can have an adverse effect on the health, safety, or welfare of people in the facility

j. free from prejudice and favoritism

Chapter 8 • Your Clinical Internship

■ Objectives

After completing this section, you will be able to:

1. Define the key terms.
2. Identify the purpose of a clinical internship.
3. List three benefits of a clinical internship.
4. Describe three ways to prepare for a clinical internship.
5. Discuss four examples of proper behavior during a clinical internship.
6. Describe three ways to ensure success during a clinical internship.
7. Explain the importance of patient confidentiality during a clinical internship.
8. Discuss the value of keeping a journal during a clinical internship.
9. Explain the importance of putting the clinical site and its patients first.
10. Describe the connection between a clinical internship and a positive reference.
11. Identify four general policies, procedures, and issues related to a successful clinical experience.

■ Directions

1. Read Chapter 8 in your textbook.
2. Complete Worksheet 1.
3. Complete Worksheet 2.
4. Complete Worksheet 3.
5. Complete Worksheet 4.
6. Complete Worksheet 5.

■ Evaluation Method

- Worksheets
- Class participation
- Section test

■ Worksheet 1

Internship Goals

In the following space, make a list of goals for your clinical internship. What are you hoping to see, to do, and to learn? What types of patients, medical procedures, and equipment do you want to experience? What questions are you hoping to get answered? What type of impression do you want to make on the site's staff?

Record the steps that you will need to take to achieve these goals. What, specifically, will you need to do to earn a positive evaluation for your internship? What attitudes, behaviors, and appearance will you need to demonstrate to begin establishing your reputation as a health care professional?

■ Worksheet 2

Pre-Internship Requirements

You are the supervisor of an outpatient clinic in your town. Your office manager has just decided to start accepting high school students for clinical internships. The students will report to you. In the space below, list five requirements that your students must meet before they begin their clinical internship in your facility.

1. _____

2. _____

3. _____

4. _____

5. _____

Internship Requirements

Continue the scenario previously presented in Worksheet 2. In the following space, list five requirements that your students must meet during their internship experience.

1. _____

2. _____

3. _____

4. _____

5. _____

Select two of your requirements and explain what you would do if students fail to meet these requirements.

1. _____

2. _____

■ Worksheet 4

Requirements for a Positive Evaluation and Reference

Continue the scenario previously presented in Worksheets 2 and 3. In the following space, list five requirements that your students must meet to obtain a positive internship evaluation from you.

1. _____

2. _____

3. _____

4. _____

5. _____

In addition to meeting these five requirements, identify three additional things that students would need to do to receive a positive reference from you.

1. _____

2. _____

3. _____

List four reasons why you would *not* give a student a positive internship evaluation or reference.

1. _____

2. _____

3. _____

4. _____

■ Worksheet 5

Matching Key Terms with Definitions

Key Terms: Match each term with its correct definition:

_____ 1. clinical internship

_____ 2. office politics

_____ 3. protocol

_____ 4. profane

_____ 5. reference

_____ 6. samples room

_____ 7. mature

_____ 8. rotation

_____ 9. penmanship

_____ 10. journal

a. a real-life learning experience obtained through working on-site in a health care facility or other setting while enrolled as a student

b. a written record of a person's thoughts and experiences

c. the ability to adjust to change

d. having reached adult development

e. clique-like relationships among groups of coworkers that involve scheming and plotting

f. handwriting

g. improper and contemptible

h. policies and procedures

i. a person who can provide information about a job applicant

j. movement from one place to another

k. a place where health care facilities keep samples of drugs and medical supplies

Chapter 9 • Health, Wellness, and Safety
Section 9.1 Health and Wellness

■ **Objectives**

After completing this section, you will be able to:

1. Define the key terms.
2. List three parts of holistic health.
3. Explain the connection between wellness and preventive care.
4. List five ways to achieve physical fitness.
5. Describe the role of alternative health care.
6. List the four functions of food when the right combination of nutrients work together in the body
7. List five basic nutrients and explain how they maintain body function.
8. Describe the USDA's MyPlate and explain its purpose.
9. Identify the characteristics of three common eating disorders.
10. List four commonly abused substances and their negative impact on the human body.
11. Give three examples of therapeutic diets.
12. Discuss why health care employers are focusing on the health and wellness of their workers.

■ **Directions**

1. Read Section 9.1 in your textbook.
2. Complete Worksheet 1.
3. Complete Worksheet 2.
4. Complete Worksheet 3.
5. Complete Worksheet 4.
6. Complete Worksheet 5.

■ **Evaluation Method**

- Worksheets
- Class participation
- Section test

Calculate Your Body Mass Index (BMI)

BMI is a number based on a person's weight and height that provides an indication of the percent of the body that is made up of fat. Because the percentage of body fat is a truer indication of health than weight alone, BMI is a useful diagnostic tool that can be used to determine if a person is overweight and by how much. BMI is an estimate of body fat. It may not be accurate for older people, or for athletes who have a greater amount of muscle mass than the average person. However, it closely tracks an average person's percentage of body fat. Use the following formula to calculate BMI:

$$\text{weight} \div \text{height}^2 \times 703 = \text{BMI}$$

For example, you would calculate the BMI for a person who weighs 150 pounds and is 5 feet 5 inches (65 inches total) tall like this: $150 \div 65^2 \times 703 = 24.96$

Next, find the BMI on this chart:

- Below 18.5   Underweight
- 18.5–24.9   Normal
- 25.0–29.9   Overweight
- 30.0 and above   Obese

This person's weight is considered normal.

Calculate your BMI using the formula. Based on this formula, are you underweight, normal weight, overweight, or obese?

In the following space, write a brief paragraph describing how this information can help you understand if you need to make lifestyle changes.

■ Worksheet 2

Calorie and Energy Requirements

Use a library or online resources to research the factors that determine a person's average calorie needs per day. Based on this information, calculate your own average daily calorie needs.

A. *The average number of calories I need per day*: _____

Using nutrition labels and other resources for calorie amounts, record your total calorie intake for three consecutive days. Pay attention to portion sizes when computing your calories.

B. *The total number of calories that I consumed per day*:

day #1 _____   day #2 _____   day #3 _____

C. *The total number of calories that I consumed over three days*: _____

Compute the average number of calories per day that you consumed. (Divide the total number of calories consumed over three days by three. For example, 9000 total calories consumed over three days would be 9000 divided by 3 for an average of 3000 calories per day.)

D. *The average number of calories that I consumed per day*: _____

Compare A (the average number of calories you need per day) with D (the average number of calories that you consumed per day).

In the following space, write a brief paragraph describing what you learned from this experience. Are you consuming too few calories, too many calories, or the right amount of calories on an average day? What, if anything, do you need to do to adjust your caloric intake? How can using this information help you become healthier?

Use a library or online resources to research the factors used to calculate Estimated Energy Requirements (EERs). These take into account your energy intake, energy expenditure, age, gender, weight, height, and physical activity level (PAL) to determine the energy requirements you need per day.

Using this information, compute your EER and record it here: _____

In the following space, write a brief paragraph indicating if you need to adjust your activity levels to meet your energy requirements and, if so, how you might do that.

■ **Worksheet 3**

Fitness and Self-Image

Review the types of fitness discussed in Section 9.1 in your textbook. Then create a list that identifies behaviors and traits that contribute to overall fitness and record your list in the following space.

Think about how your fitness affects your self-image. In the space below, note the behaviors and traits that can lead to a positive self-image or a negative self-image. Comment on any improvements that you might wish to make.

■ Worksheet 4

My Profile

In the following space, create a profile of yourself, including your height, weight, and activity level. Include your BMI, daily calorie needs, EER, and fitness self-image notes.

Use MyPlate to plan a healthy one-day menu for yourself. Include meals, snacks, and beverages and the appropriate number of servings required to meet your personal calorie needs. Include essential nutrients (proteins, carbohydrates, fats, minerals, vitamins, and water). Be sure to consult nutrition labels for information about the nutrients found in the foods you are including in your menu. When the day's menu is complete, follow that menu for a day. In the following space, record what you have learned from this experience. Do you plan to make any changes? Why or why not?

List three things you could do to improve your overall health and wellness.

1. _____

2. _____

3. _____

What might prevent you from accomplishing your goals, and how can you overcome these barriers?

Matching Key Terms with Definitions

Key Terms #1: Match each term with its correct definition:

_____ 1. calorie

_____ 2. aerobic

_____ 3. carbohydrates

_____ 4. cosmetic

_____ 5. deficiency

_____ 6. digestion

_____ 7. body mass index

_____ 8. addiction

_____ 9. cholesterol

_____ 10. bingeing

_____ 11. amino acids

_____ 12. cellulose

_____ 13. absorption

a. to take up liquid or other matter

b. a compulsion to continue using a substance even though it has negative consequences

c. requiring oxygen

d. compounds found in living cells that contain carbon, oxygen, hydrogen, and nitrogen and join together to form proteins

e. eating or drinking excessively

f. measure of body fat based on height and weight for adult men and women

g. unit of measure of the fuel value of food

h. groups of organic compounds that include sugars, starches, celluloses, and gums that provide major sources of energy

i. the primary component of plant cell walls which provides the fiber and bulk necessary for optimal functioning of the digestive tract

j. a type of lipid or fat found in the body; produced by the liver or eaten in food

k. something done for the sake of appearance

l. a disease caused by lack of a nutrient

m. when waste matter is discharged from the blood, tissues, or organs

n. the process of making food absorbable by dissolving it and breaking it down into simpler chemical compounds that occur in the living body chiefly through the action of enzymes secreted into the alimentary canal

Key Terms #2: Match each term with its correct definition:

_____ 1. excreted

_____ 2. hemoglobin

_____ 3. malnutrition

_____ 4. infirmity

_____ 5. minerals

_____ 6. nutrients

_____ 7. lactation

_____ 8. metabolism

_____ 9. metabolize

_____ 10. invincible

_____ 11. essential

_____ 12. health risk
assessments

_____ 13. fats

a. necessary

b. when waste matter is discharged from the blood, tissues, or organs

c. groups of organic compounds that, together with carbohydrates and proteins, constitute the primary structural material of living cells; also known as lipids

d. questionnaires that identify which health issues a person needs to focus on based on his or her medical history and lifestyle

e. complex chemical in the blood; carries oxygen and carbon dioxide

f. unsound or unhealthy state of being

g. incapable of being overcome

h. the body's process of producing milk to feed newborn babies

i. poor nutrition caused by an insufficient or poorly balanced diet or by a medical condition

j. collection of chemical reactions that takes place in the body's cells to convert the fuel in food into energy

k. to break down substances in cells to obtain energy

l. inorganic elements that occur in nature; essential to every cell

m. chemical compounds found in food

n. responding to something that has happened

Key Terms #3: Match each term with its correct definition:

_____ 1. resistance

_____ 2. purging

_____ 3. self-image

_____ 4. vitamins

_____ 5. vitality

_____ 6. reactive

_____ 7. screenings

_____ 8. toxicity

_____ 9. taboos

_____ 10. proteins

_____ 11. regulate

_____ 12. proactive

a. anticipating and acting in advance

b. complex compounds found in plant and animal tissue, essential for heat, energy, and growth

c. causing oneself to vomit

d. responding to something that has happened

e. to control or adjust

f. the ability of the body to protect itself from disease

g. tests or examinations that are done to find a disease or condition before symptoms appear

h. the mental picture that a person has of himself or herself

i. to break down substances in cells to obtain energy

j. banned from social custom

k. a disease caused by too much of a nutrient

l. the ability of an organism to go on living

m. groups of substances necessary for normal functioning and maintenance of health

Section 9.2 Infection Control and Safety at Work

■ Objectives

After completing this section, you will be able to:

1. Define the key terms.
2. Differentiate between *pathogenic* and *nonpathogenic* microorganisms.
3. List five ways to prevent the spread of microorganisms and viruses.
4. Define *medical asepsis* and list five aseptic techniques.
5. List three ways by which bloodborne diseases are accidentally passed.
6. Describe the purpose of Universal Precautions.
7. Define *OSHA* and explain the agency's role in safety.
8. Explain the health care worker's role in maintaining a safe workplace.
9. Identify five general safety rules.
10. Identify what you are responsible for knowing and doing when a disaster occurs.
11. List the three elements required to start a fire, and four ways to prevent fires.
12. List six rules of correct body mechanics.
13. Demonstrate the correct techniques for lifting and moving objects.

■ Directions

1. Read Section 9.2 in your textbook.
2. Complete Worksheet 1.
3. Complete Worksheet 2.
4. Complete Worksheet 3.
5. Complete Worksheet 4.
6. Complete Worksheet 5.

■ Evaluation Method

- Worksheets
- Class participation
- Section test

Super Bugs

The scientific and medical communities are constantly finding new information about how microorganisms affect our lives. This constant flow of new information makes it necessary to research how new findings affect us. Conduct some research in a library or online to identify a *super bug* of interest to researchers. In the space below, describe its nature, its appearance, and its pattern of growth. How does this superbug affect the body? What symptoms does it cause? How does it spread? What precautions can be taken to protect against infection?

■ Worksheet 2

OSHA Standards

Using a library or online resources, research OSHA standards for workplace safety. In the following space, record five OSHA procedures that relate to safety in health care facilities.

1.

2.

3.

4.

5.

■ Worksheet 3

Infection Control and Prevention

Indentify two infections that could spread throughout your school. In the following space, record the name of each infection. Explain the source of the infection and how it spreads. Describe the steps your school should take to prevent the infection from occurring. Describe the steps your school should take to treat the infection if it occurs.

Infection #1:

Infection #2:

Share this information with your classmates and teacher. Combine this information from all of the students into one Master List. In the following space, describe how this Master List could be shared with everyone in your school to prevent the spread of infections.

School Safety and Preparedness

Divide into five teams. Each team will complete one of the following assignments:

1. Develop a safety plan for your school.

2. Develop a disaster plan for your school.

3. Develop a bioterrorism plan for your school.

4. Develop a fire safety and fire response plan for your school.

5. Develop an ergonomics plan for your school.

Each plan should include the following:

a. Purpose or goal of the plan

b. Why the plan is necessary

c. Who should comply with the plan

d. The steps, precautions, and procedures that need to be followed

e. How the plan could be evaluated to measure its effectiveness

f. What equipment, training, and resources would be required to implement the plan

After each team has developed a plan, work with your teacher to find out which plans already exist for your school. Compare these existing plans with your plans, and note any differences. In the following space, describe how these approaches to *safety at school* could be applied to *safety in health care facilities.*

■ Worksheet 5

Matching Key Terms with Definitions

Key Terms #1: Match each term with its correct definition:

_____ 1. autoclaves	a. side by side
_____ 2. ambulate	b. keeping the body in proper position—in a straight line without twisting
_____ 3. bacteriostatic	c. walk
_____ 4. bacteria	d. able to grow and function without oxygen
_____ 5. biohazard	e. sterile condition, free from all germs
_____ 6. aseptic technique	f. method used to make the environment, the worker, and the patient as germ-free as possible
_____ 7. bactericidal	g. sterilizers that use steam under pressure to kill all forms of bacteria on objects that pathogens live on and can transfer infection
_____ 8. bloodborne	h. a disease-causing microorganism
_____ 9. alignment	i. not disease-causing
_____ 10. abreast	j. kills bacteria
_____ 11. asepsis	k. slows or stops the growth of bacteria
_____ 12. anaerobic	l. biological materials or infectious agents that may cause harm to human, animal, or environmental health
	m. carried in the blood

Key Terms #2: Match each term with its correct definition:

_____ 1. chain of infection
_____ 2. disinfection
_____ 3. ergonomic
_____ 4. generalized
_____ 5. gait belt
_____ 6. feces
_____ 7. flammable
_____ 8. frayed
_____ 9. contaminated
_____ 10. enterotoxin
_____ 11. decompose
_____ 12. crouch

a. a chain of events, all interconnected, is required for an infection to spread

b. soiled, unclean, not suitable for use

c. to stoop, using the large muscles of the legs to help maintain balance

d. to decay, to break down

e. process of freeing from microorganisms by physical or chemical means

f. poisonous substance that is produced in, or originates in, the contents of the intestine

g. an object or practice designed to reduce injury

h. solid waste that is evacuated from the body through the anus; also known as stools

i. catches fire easily or burns quickly

j. worn or tattered; such as electrical cords may be worn, causing wires to be exposed

k. a safety device used to move a patient from one place to another; also used to help hold up a weak person while he or she walks

l. affecting all of the body

m. affecting one area of the body

Key Terms #3: Match each term with its correct definition:

_____ 1. gravity

_____ 2. nonpathogenic

_____ 3. host

_____ 4. localized

_____ 5. mandates

_____ 6. nosocomial infection

_____ 7. parasites

_____ 8. pathogenic

_____ 9. horseplay

_____ 10. observant

_____ 11. load

_____ 12. hazards

a. natural force or pull toward the earth; in the body, the center of gravity is usually the center of the body

b. things that may cause harm to human, animal, or environmental health

c. rowdy and childish behavior; acting inappropriately in a work environment

d. the organism from which a microorganism takes nourishment; the microorganism gives nothing in return and causes disease or illness

e. kills bacteria

f. weight of an object or person that is to be moved

g. affecting one area of the body

h. orders or commands

i. not disease-causing

j. an infection acquired while in a health care setting, such as a hospital

k. quick to see and understand

l. organisms obtaining nourishment from other organisms they are living in or on

m. disease-causing

Key Terms #4: Match each term with its correct definition:

_____ 1. protist

_____ 2. salmonella

_____ 3. saprophytes

_____ 4. sterilized

_____ 5. susceptible

_____ 6. spirochetes

_____ 7. Standard Precautions

_____ 8. Universal Precautions

_____ 9. transmitting

_____ 10. viruses

_____ 11. toxins

_____ 12. shock

_____ 13. rickettsiae

a.   an organism belonging to the kingdom that includes protozoans, bacteria, and single-celled algae and fungi

b.   parasitic microorganisms that live on another living organism and cause disease

c.   a rod-shaped bacterium found in the intestine that can cause food poisoning, gastroenteritis, and typhoid fever

d.   organisms that live on dead organic matter

e.   convulsion of muscles and extreme stimulation of nerves when an electric current passes through the body

f.   slender, coil-shaped organisms

g.   guidelines designed to reduce the risk of transmission of microorganisms from recognized and unrecognized sources of infection in the hospital

h.   made free from all living organisms

i.   capable of being affected or infected; the body can be attacked by microorganisms and become ill

j.   poisonous substances

k.   causing to go from one person to another person

l.   a set of precautions that prevents the transmission of HIV, HBV, HCV, and other bloodborne pathogens when providing health care

m.   genetic material that is surrounded by a protective coat and that can only reproduce inside a host cell; can only be seen under a microscope

n.   things that may cause harm to human, animal, or environmental health

Chapter 10 • Employment, Leadership, and Professional Development

Section 10.1 Employment Skills

■ **Objectives**

After completing this section, you will be able to:

1. Define the key terms.
2. List three sources of information on job openings.
3. Describe four characteristics of a professional résumé.
4. Name five things you should do when filling out a job application form.
5. Explain why employers use pre-employment assessments.
6. Describe five ways to present a professional image during a job interview.
7. Discuss the difference between *traditional* and *behavioral* interview questions.
8. List three ways to convince interviewers that you are serious about wanting the job.
9. Describe what you should do if you don't get a job offer.
10. Discuss the role of compromising to eventually get the job you want.

■ **Directions**

1. Read Section 10.1 in your textbook.
2. Complete Worksheet 1.
3. Complete Worksheet 2.
4. Complete Worksheet 3.
5. Complete Worksheet 4.
6. Complete Worksheet 5.

■ **Evaluation Method**

- Worksheets
- Class participation
- Section test

■ Worksheet 1

Analyzing the Job Market

Analyze the job market for the health care profession you plan to pursue. Review current labor trends and future projections. Is there an oversupply or a shortage of these workers? What factors are influencing these trends and projections? In the following space, write a brief report describing how these trends may impact the job market when you are ready to launch your job search.

■ Worksheet 2

My Résumé

Using the information in your textbook, develop your résumé. If you already have a résumé, review the document, update it, and make whatever improvements it requires based on what you've learned. Include all of your important information and make sure the document is well organized and professional in appearance. Exchange résumés with a classmate and offer suggestions for improvement. Be sure to include a copy of your résumé in your career portfolio and keep your résumé up to date.

My Cover Letter

Write a cover letter to accompany your résumé. Address the letter to the Director of Human Resources at a local health care organization in your community. State that you are available to begin employment upon graduation from your health care educational program, and identify the position in which you are interested. Exchange cover letters with a classmate and offer suggestions for improvement. After making improvements, include a copy of your cover letter in your career portfolio for future reference.

■ Worksheet 4

My Interview

In the following space, list ten questions that you would expect to be asked during a job interview. List your answer for each question. Also list three items from your career portfolio (other than your résumé) that you would take with you to the job interview in case you have an opportunity to present them.

Interview Questions and Answers:

1. Question:

Answer:

2. Question:

Answer:

3. Question:

Answer:

4. Question:

Answer:

5. Question:

Answer:

6. Question:

Answer:

7. Question:

Answer:

8. Question:

Answer:

9. Question:

Answer:

10. Question:

Answer:

Career portfolio items to take to my interview:

1.

2.

3.

Matching Key Terms with Definitions

Key Terms #1: Match each term with its correct definition:

_____ 1. behavioral questions

_____ 2. blogs

_____ 3. credit report

_____ 4. employment benefits

_____ 5. citations

_____ 6. employment agencies

_____ 7. discriminate

_____ 8. cover letter

a. ask how you *did* behave in certain situations

b. similar to newspaper columns but published on the Internet instead of in print

c. extra compensation for accepting a job offer

d. honorable mention for receiving an outcome or result

e. letter introducing a job applicant to a potential employer

f. a review of records to assess a person's financial status

g. to treat a person or group unfairly on the basis of prejudice

h. companies that connect job applicants with employers

i. employer-paid insurance and retirement savings

Key Terms #2: Match each term with its correct definition:

_____ 1. job application

_____ 2. networking

_____ 3. official transcript

_____ 4. occupational preferences

_____ 5. employment status

_____ 6. hire-on bonus

_____ 7. human resources department

a. to remain constant to a purpose

b. hired to work full-time, part-time, or supplemental

c. extra compensation for accepting a job offer

d. current term for personnel department

e. form used to apply for a job; also known as an employment application

f. interacting with a variety of people in different settings

g. the types of work and work settings that you prefer

h. grade report that is printed, sealed, and mailed directly to the recipient to prevent tampering by the applicant

Key Terms #3: Match each term with its correct definition:

_____ 1. résumé

_____ 2. retention

_____ 3. screen

_____ 4. vested

_____ 5. personnel department

_____ 6. selection process

_____ 7. traditional questions

_____ 8. retirement benefits

_____ 9. pre-employment assessments

_____ 10. perseverance

a. ask how you *did* behave in certain situations

b. to remain constant to a purpose

c. people within an organization who recruit, select, and employ job applicants

d. tests and other instruments used to measure knowledge, skills, and personality traits

e. document summarizing job qualifications

f. the process of keeping

g. employer-funded pension contributions

h. to sift, filter, or separate

i. steps to determine which applicants are chosen

j. ask how you *would* behave in certain situations

k. fully enrolled in, and eligible for, benefits

Section 10.2 Leadership Skills and Professional Development

■ Objectives

After completing this section, you will be able to:

1. Define the key terms.
2. Explain why effective leadership is crucial in health care.
3. Describe four characteristics of effective leaders.
4. Identify three ways to develop leadership skills.
5. List two benefits of participating in a health care professional association.
6. Describe the goals and role of HOSA.
7. Explain why health care workers must be lifelong learners.
8. Describe five resources for professional development.
9. Discuss the benefits of having a career plan.
10. Explain how succession planning creates opportunities for job advancement.

■ Directions

1. Read Section 10.2 in your textbook.
2. Complete Worksheet 1.
3. Complete Worksheet 2.
4. Complete Worksheet 3.
5. Complete Worksheet 4.
6. Complete Worksheet 5.

■ Evaluation Method

- Worksheets
- Class participation
- Section test

■ Worksheet 1

An Effective Leader

Identify a leader whom you respect and admire. This could be someone whom you know personally, such as an athletic coach, teacher, supervisor, or a leader in your church or community. This could also be a leader on a state, national, or international level—someone whom you don't know personally but respect and admire.

In the following space, write the leader's name and indicate how you know about this person. Write a brief paragraph describing why you view this person as an effective leader. Include personal and professional characteristics, evidence of leadership skills, and examples of the results that he or she obtains.

Selecting the Best Leader

You are the chief executive officer of a small hospital in a Western U.S. state. You have a key leadership position to fill and have received applications from more than 50 people who appear to meet the minimum requirements for the job.

In the following space, list the five most important qualifications you would seek to find the best applicant for the job. Then list five interview questions that you would ask to evaluate the leadership skills of the finalists for the position.

Qualifications:

1. _____

2. _____

3. _____

4. _____

5. _____

Interview Questions:

1. _____

2. _____

3. _____

4. _____

5. _____

■ Worksheet 3

Career Goals

In the following space, list three SMART goals for the first phase of your health career—goals that you expect to achieve within the next three years. For each goal, list at least one step you will need to complete to accomplish your goal.

SMART goals for the first phase of my career:

1. _____

2. _____

3. _____

Steps to achieve my first-phase career goals:

Goal #1 _____

Goal #2 _____

Goal #3 _____

List three SMART goals for the next phase of your health career—goals you expect to achieve within the next eight years. For each goal, list at least one step you will need to complete to accomplish your goal.

SMART goals for the next phase of my career:

4. _____

5. _____

6. _____

Steps to achieve my next-phase career goals:

Goal #4 _____

Goal #5 _____

Goal #6 _____

When Career Goals Change

Consider each of the six career goals that you listed in Worksheet 3. In the following space, list at least six factors that might cause you to change some, or all, of your career goals. Consider factors such as barriers (insufficient funds to attend college, the place where you want to work isn't hiring), changes in your personal life (marriage, relocation to a new town), and unexpected career opportunities (job openings due to worker retirements, the requirement to undergo cross-training).

Factors that might cause me to change my career goals:

1. _____

2. _____

3. _____

4. _____

5. _____

6. _____

In the space below, write a brief paragraph about the need to be flexible and adaptive to change when making career plans.

■ Worksheet 5

Matching Key Terms with Definitions

Key Terms #1: Match each term with its correct definition:

_____ 1. clocking in and out

_____ 2. dynamic

_____ 3. static

_____ 4. legislative issues

_____ 5. extemporaneous

_____ 6. work commitment

a. using a time clock or electronic system to record hours worked

b. in motion, energetic and vigorous

c. stationary and motionless

d. spoken without preparation or notes

e. topics involving local, state, and national law-making

f. existing as a possibility

g. a written agreement to work for an employer for a specified period of time

Key Terms #2: Match each term with its correct definition:

_____ 1. morale

_____ 2. perks

_____ 3. tuition assistance

_____ 4. reactionary

_____ 5. potential

_____ 6. succession planning

_____ 7. professional development

a. the mental or emotional spirit of a person or a group

b. benefits that come with status

c. stationary and motionless

d. existing as a possibility

e. education for people who have begun their careers and need to continue growing

f. responding to a stimulus or influence

g. a proactive approach to identifying and preparing employees to fill positions when other workers retire

h. paying for a portion of college tuition fees

Closing Thoughts

■ Directions

1. Read Closing Thoughts in your textbook.

2. Complete Worksheet 1.

3. Complete Worksheet 2.

4. Complete Worksheet 3.

5. Complete Worksheet 4.

6. Complete Worksheet 5.

■ Evaluation Method

- Worksheets
- Class participation

■ Worksheet 1

Changes in My Life

List three of the changes that you are undergoing, or about to undergo, in your life.

1. _____

2. _____

3. _____

In the space below, write a paragraph that explains how change can be a good thing if you anticipate change and are well prepared for it. Discuss how your future can be *exciting* and *scary* at the same time. Refer to this quote by journalist Edgar Ansel Mowrer: "Life is unsafe at any speed, and therein lies much of its fascination."

Twenty Things to Do

Review the following list of *Twenty Things to Do*. Select five of the items and circle them. On the next page, write one example of what you will do to comply with five of the *Twenty Things to Do* that you selected.

1. Choose your occupation and your career carefully.
2. Conduct occupational research, monitor labor trends and projections, and consider your personal values, interests, motivations, personality traits, and knowledge, skills, and abilities to find the perfect career match for you.
3. Have a plan and expect it to change.
4. Know where you're headed and how you're going to get there.
5. Expect things to change, but stay on the right track and take advantage of unexpected opportunities when they arise.
6. Keep your SMART goals up-to-date and share them with people who can help you succeed.
7. Set yourself up for success.
8. Use good judgment and make thoughtful decisions.
9. Build your resources and your network of supporters.
10. When you need some help, don't hesitate to ask for it.
11. Don't let other people discourage you or prevent you from reaching your goals.
12. If your goals are worth achieving, they're worth fighting for, so hang in there.
13. Keep an optimistic attitude and surround yourself with people who have a positive influence on your life.
14. Keep your priorities straight; place your job and your career high on your list.
15. Make your health and wellness and your commitment to spending quality time with family and friends high priorities.
16. Demonstrate reliability, dependability, accountability, and trustworthiness as the keys to earning self-respect and the respect of others.
17. Never stop learning; always be a student.
18. Continually sharpen your skills, maintain your competence, and participate in continuing education every chance that you get.
19. Remember that knowledge is the key to just about everything.
20. Develop your leadership skills; articulate a vision and make it a reality through collaboration with others.

Examples of what I will do to comply with five of the *Twenty Things to Do:*

1.

2.

3.

4.

5.

Five Things to Think About and Remember

Review the following list of *Five Things to Think About and Remember.* On the next page, write one example of what you will do to comply with each of these *Five Things to Think About and Remember.*

1. *Who you are as a person makes a difference.* If you want to be seen by others as a professional, you must earn and maintain that honor every day that you

   come to work. Demonstrating a strong work ethic, meeting legal and ethical responsibilities, and displaying character traits that reflect compassion and respect for others are the keys to a professional reputation. Represent your employer with dignity, pride, and loyalty. Always *do the right thing* because *it's the right thing to do.*

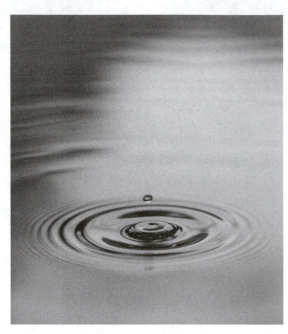

Source: Nejron Photo/Shutterstock

2. *It's all about the patient.* When you work in health care, it's not about you or your job title or your schedule for the day. It's always about the patient. How your patients feel about their health care experience can have a significant impact on the success of your organization. *High tech* drives advancement in health care and medicine, but it can never replace the importance of *high touch.*

3. *Care about quality and safety.* Health care is an extremely complex industry with life and death literally hanging in the balance. It's easy for things to *fall through the cracks* and cause problems. Pay attention to details and find ways to improve quality of care. Help create and maintain an environment where patients, coworkers, and others feel safe and *in good hands.*

4. *Keep up with current events.* This is your career, so be aware of what's going on in the health care industry, in your profession, and in your place of employment. Get involved and help shape the future.

5. *Make positive ripples with everything you say and do.* Stop and think before you act. Be present in the moment, and act with intention and self-awareness. Consider the impact that your attitude, appearance, and behavior have on other people. Respect other people's opinions and values, and do your best to improve the lives of those around you.

Examples of how I will comply with each of these *Five Things to Think About and Remember:*

1.

2.

3.

4.

5.

Three Next Steps

Review the following list of *Three Next Steps*. In the space below the list, write one example of what you will do to comply with each of these *Three Next Steps*.

1. *Complete your education.* If you decide to focus on just one goal right now, make it "to graduate." You'll need a strong academic foundation upon which to build your career and your future. It all starts with earning good grades and completing your education.

2. *Develop your skills.* Focus on your soft skills as well as your hard skills. Improve your ability to communicate, resolve conflict, and solve problems through critical thinking. Hone your computer skills and your ability to manage your time, personal finances, and stress. Learn to appreciate and accept people who are different from you. Embrace diversity and find ways to make it work for you and for the people around you.

3. *Accept responsibility.* Adopt the attitude, "the buck stops here." Make your own decisions with the support of your family and friends, and then accept the consequences. Admit when you've made a mistake and learn from it. This is your life, so seize control of it. Take some calculated risks to stretch a bit and develop your full potential. When the going gets rough, hang in there.

Examples of how I will comply with each of these *Three Next Steps:*

1.

2.

3.

It's Really Up To You

You will soon become the *Chief Executive Officer of Your Life*. You can start preparing now by making the right decisions, for the right reasons, at the right times. The time you spend now planning for your future will be time well invested. It's really up to you.

Complete the following checklist:

_____ I have researched health care occupations, and I am sure that a health career is a good match for me.

_____ I have given careful thought to my future, and I have the support of my family and other key people in my life.

_____ I have the courage and the motivation it takes to tackle and overcome tough challenges.

_____ I am serious about serving the needs of others and making a difference in their lives as well as my own.

_____ I am going to become a health care professional and make a difference.

In the following space, write a paragraph that answers the question, "Where will you fit in?"

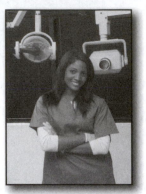

Source: OLJ Studio/Shutterstock

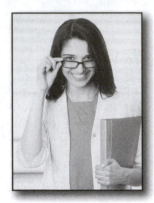

Source: Konstantin Chagin/
Shutterstock

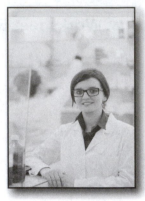

Source: shock/Shutterstock

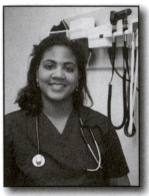

Source: Rob Marmion/
Shutterstock

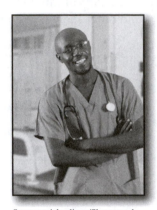

Source: michaeljung/Shutterstock

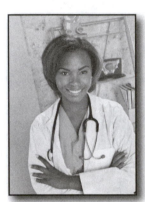

Source: REDAV/Shutterstock

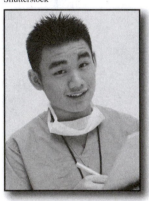

Source: Blend Images/Shutterstock

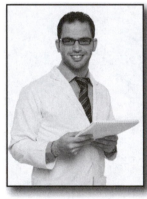

Source: Ebtikar/Shutterstock

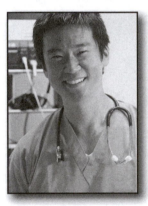

Source: James Peragine/
Shutterstock

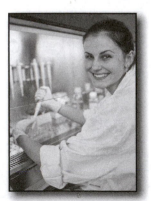

Source: lightpoet/Shutterstock

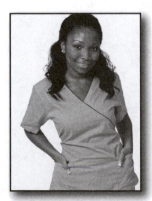

Source: Aspen Photo/Shutterstock

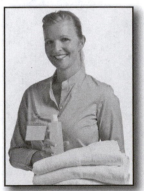

Source: AVAVA/Shutterstock

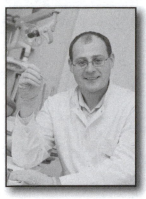

Source: Dmitry Kalinovsky/
Shutterstock

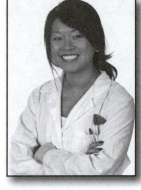

Source: aceshot1/Shutterstock

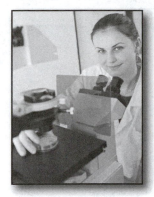

Source: lightpoet/Shutterstock

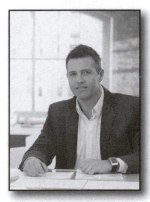

Source: Tyler Olson/Shutterstock

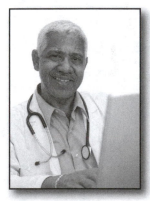

Source: Elnur/Shutterstock

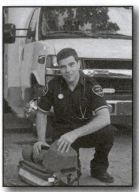

Source: StockLite/Shutterstock

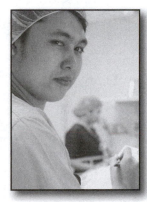

Source: pedalist/Shutterstock

Source: Rob Marmion/
Shutterstock

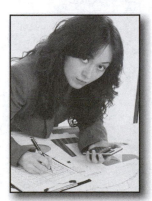

Source: Zadorozhnyi Viktor/
Shutterstock

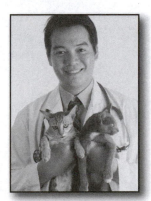

Source: william casey/Shutterstock

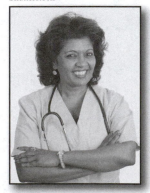

Source: Lisa F. Young/
Shutterstock

NOTES

NOTES

NOTES

NOTES

NOTES

NOTES

NOTES